Discovering

*Pure Classical **Pilates***

Theory and Practice as Joseph Pilates Intended
The Traditional Method vs. The Lies for Sale

Peter Fiasca, Ph.D.

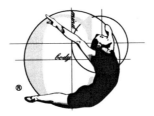

Discovering Pure Classical **Pilates**
Theory and Practice as Joseph Pilates Intended
The Traditional Method vs. The Lies for Sale

Second American Edition 2009

Discovering Pure Classical Pilates can be
purchased at www.ClassicalPilates.net.
We offer a special price discount for ordering 10+ books.

Library of Congress Control Number: 2008943231

ISBN 10: 0-6152-4562-5

ISBN 13: 978-0-6152456-2-1

Art Design: John Weir
Photography: Richard Quindry, Beth Clarke, Lauren Diamond & Dan Demetriad
Front Cover Instructors: Sandy Shimoda and Peter Fiasca
Back Cover Instructors: Christina Gloger and Peter Fiasca

Infinite thanks to Christina Gloger, Steve Hash, Junghee Kallander,
Jim Monroe, Sandy Shimoda and Jamie Trout for their extraordinary work
in the series of six Classical Pilates Technique DVDs and for expertly
demonstrating the traditional Pilates exercises included in this book.

Caution:
This book is not intended for treatment of any injuries.
Do not use as a replacement for medical care.
Obtain a physician's advice before starting any physical fitness program.

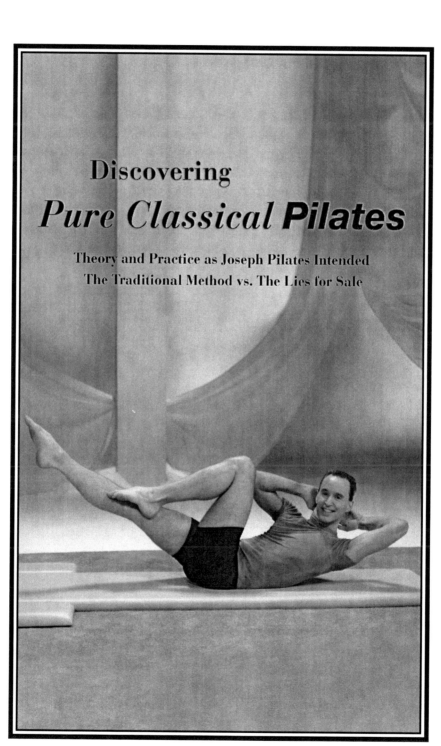

Discovering

Pure Classical **Pilates**

Theory and Practice as Joseph Pilates Intended
The Traditional Method vs. The Lies for Sale

Dedication

This book is dedicated to Joseph and Clara Pilates, as well as to my primary teachers, Romana Kryzanowska and Jay Grimes, who have preserved the full spectrum of Contrology with love, wisdom, and a wonderful sense of humor. It is equally important to acknowledge all the loyal, exceptionally skilled professionals who share their knowledge of Joseph Pilates' traditional method with students and future generations of faithful instructors.

Contents

Chapter 1
Pure Classical Pilates Overture
My Journey and
The Passion for Preservation 1

Chapter 2
Pure Classical Pilates Inside & Out...................9
   Foundations and Beginning the Journey...........................10
   The "7 Cs" of Pure Classical Pilates 15
   Joseph Pilates' Periodic Table of Elements........................18
   Pure Classical Pilates is Not Physical Therapy.................20
   Pure Classical Pilates is Not Yoga......................................21
   Pure Classical Pilates is Not Dance 25
   Faithfulness to Technique 29
   The Educational Art of Teaching Pilates............................30
   The Apparatus..34

Chapter 3
Joseph Pilates:
The Making of the Master and His Work 37
   Pilates and Paideia...38
   A Balancing Act Between the Mind and Body..................43
   The Spiritual Dimension of
   Joseph Pilates' Traditional Method 53

Chapter 4
Four Necessary Conditions of Joseph Pilates' Traditional method 61

The Flat-Back Position....................................62

External Rotation as the Standard 70

The "Ins and Outs" of Proper Breathing 73

Fine Art of the Flow 80

Chapter 5
The Body and Mind 89

The Traditional Method and Life Lessons:
Metaphors for Living.....................................90

Pure Classical Pilates & Psychology:
Similarities and Differences.............................92

Psychological Defense Trends Reflected in Pilates 98

Links Between Psychology and Pure Classical Pilates..102

The Pure Classical Pilates Studio:
An Interpersonal Learning Lab 111

Nonverbal Communication as
Unconscious or Implied Meaning 114

Chapter 6
Roadblocks to the Pure Classical Experience

Small Business, Big Business and Rewriting Tradition 119

The Great Debate:
Trust The Master or Mess with Perfection 120

The Great Decline:
Derivative Styles of the Traditional Method.................125

Pilates for Profit: The Price of Marketplace Mutation ...133

Professions and Professional Membership 141

Gender Imbalance yet Equal Opportunity.....................146

Chapter 7
Keeping the Tradition Alive 153
The Worldwide Academy of Traditionalists 155
Let It Be: Rewriting Tradition Rewards No One 158
Pure Classical Pilates on Film:
A Quest to Capture the Magic...............................161
Proclaiming the Importance of
Joseph Pilates' Traditional Work................................164

Chapter 8
Standards of Excellence, Studio Conduct, Basic Tips and a Proposed Code Of Ethics....167
Conduct in the Traditional Studio 168
The Ideal World Checklist:
Pure Classical Pilates Do's and Don'ts...........................171
Pure Classical Pilates: A Proposed Code of Ethics 173

Epilogue..179
A Call for a Return to the Classics 180
Fanning the Flame:
The Future of Pure Classical Pilates 183

References 186

Appendix 190
Academy Directory...190
A Pure Classical Collection:
The Principles Come to Life on DVD................................191

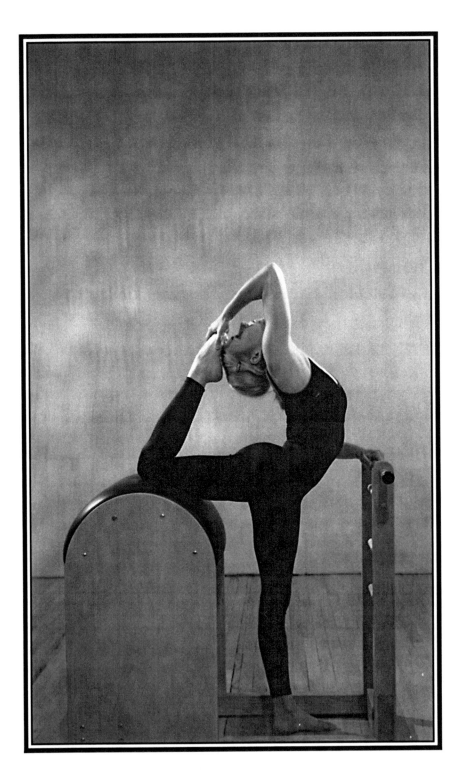

Chapter 1

Pure Classical Pilates Overture

My Journey and The Passion for Preservation

Chapter One

Discovering Pure Classical Pilates is not a "how-to" manual of Joseph Pilates' exercises and workouts. It is not my intention to provide descriptions of exercises, nor is it my intention to replace consistent study with a well-trained and dedicated traditional instructor. Instead, I offer you an explanation of the foundations and the benefits of Pure Classical Pilates — with the concerned hope of retaining its purity and integrity for generations to come.

Discovering Pure Classical Pilates looks deeply into Joseph Pilates' traditional method of mental and physical conditioning by describing its foundations, goals, movement qualities and benefits. Specific attention is given to the ways in which market forces, individual creativity or ambition lead to deterioration and commercialization of the traditional Pilates method. This book harkens back in time to Joseph Pilates' own two books — *Your Health* (1934) and *Return to Life Through Contrology* (1945) — by exploring social, economic, psychological and spiritual issues associated with his traditional work. There is so much more to *Discovering Pure Classical Pilates!* Within this book, you will uncover the passionate and priceless treasures found only in the historically accurate technique as taught by traditionalists throughout the world.

Although Joseph Pilates' traditional method of body conditioning provides optimal strength, flexibility, energetic vitality and balanced muscular precision for everyday movement and athletic activity, the deviations and mutations of his traditional work now flooding the marketplace do not. This book explains why we must preserve the historically accurate Pilates method before it becomes so watered down that it is in danger of being forever lost. I encourage students and teachers alike to learn more about this remarkable man and the traditional method he called Contrology — the complete coordination of body, mind and spirit. Joseph Pilates fundamentally believed that Contrology helps prevent and fight disease by strengthening the body's immune system.

Why use the term *Pure Classical Pilates*? Because modern deviations from Joseph Pilates' traditional method run rampant throughout the profession, and sometimes they are incorrectly — or falsely — labeled "classical Pilates." It is, therefore, important to make a clear distinction between these counterfeit approaches and Joseph Pilates' traditional technique. As you embark on your journey through *Discovering Pure Classical Pilates*, keep these key points in mind:

- *There is only one Pure Classical Pilates -*
   Joseph Pilates' traditional method.
- *There are many derivative approaches incorrectly*
   or falsely called Pilates.
- *"Contemporary Pilates" is a contradiction in terms.*

It has been over twenty years since I discovered the Pilates method. Originally, I came to it to heal an old knee injury. When I decided to try Pilates — admittedly, after some procrastination — I was very fortunate to find Wee-Tai Hom's studio at 160 E. 56th Street in New York City. At the time, This studio is where Romana Kryzanowska shared her wealth of knowledge and decades of experience working directly with Joseph Pilates. Romana would sometimes describe the traditional method as a science of the body and an art form. She also likened the work to "poetry in motion." Because of her extensive work with the master, Romana is considered by traditionalists as the world-renowned protégé of Joseph Pilates. We also consider protégé Jay Grimes in the same realm because of his extensive training with Joseph and Clara Pilates over the years and because Jay preserves the traditional method with deep insight, high intelligence and good humor.

At the beginning of my studies, Wee-Tai Hom's studio was the world's foremost educational and training center preserving Joseph Pilates' traditional method. I signed up for my first ten lessons, basically on faith. Phoebe Higgins, my first teacher, had studied with Romana since the age of fourteen. Phoebe taught with charm and wit, while simultaneously expecting the same intense and precise work that is integral to Joseph Pilates' traditional system.

Modern deviations of Joseph Pilates' traditional system run rampant throughout the profession.

The exercises were challenging, to say the least! In particular, I found Mat exercises somewhat frustrating, because my body could not "comprehend" the movement very well. Eventually, however, it was these repeated Mat exercises—and apparatus workouts—that helped my body gradually discover proper placement and correct movement patterns. Over time, the work became more familiar, and I began to experience the benefits from this extraordinary system of mental and physical health.

I was so excited with the new positive changes traditional Pilates was bringing to my body and mind that I nearly quit my academic schooling at the time to immediately begin training as a traditional instructor! You see, I was on another journey — working toward a Ph.D. in psychology. So, while I remained committed on my chosen path, Pilates was relegated to the time between studying and my work at a Philadelphia hospital.

Yet, the benefits and pleasures of Joseph Pilates' tradition kept tugging at me. The more I studied and practiced the traditional method, the more I understood how genuinely wonderful it was for my physical and mental health. I had better energy, enhanced mental focus, faster reflexes, improved coordination, taller posture and something strangely new — flexible strength.

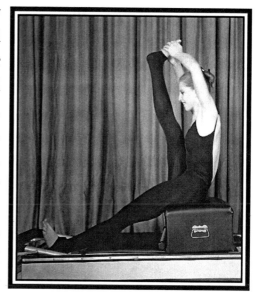

In contrast to the tight sinew strength I gained from weight training, or the straightforward endurance I achieved from jogging, Pure Classical Pilates helped heal my knee injury while increasing stamina and flexible strength. Yet there were other benefits that exceeded the physical ones. Because the traditional work has varied and complex movements, achieving correct muscular effort, coordination, articulation and flow necessitates intelligence and mental discipline.

Chapter One

I truly had the sense of *accomplishing a workout* instead of *drudging through a workout*. Also, I noticed my temperament was gradually changing because I didn't let everyday circumstances cause frustration so easily. I seemed to be more accepting of myself and, in general, more patient. Given these physical, mental and spiritual benefits, it was not surprising that I craved the movement of Joseph Pilates' traditional technique. *The work simply helped me feel so much better, and it continues to do so today.*

After completing the apprenticeship program with Romana in 1998, I continued teaching part-time at The Pilates Studio in New York City, as well as at my home studio in Pennsylvania. Before long, I realized that while psychology may have been my first calling—it was not my life-long calling. And though it was not an easy decision to leave my job as a psychologist, with its benefits and spacious office with a view, I knew it was my only decision. After much consideration, I began doing the work I was born to do, teaching Pure Classical Pilates. It was a decision I've yet to regret for even one moment.

Today, I feel a sense of urgency to help preserve the traditional method, saving it from being forever diluted by a marketing industry intent on continuous reinvention. From 2002-2006 I developed a series of DVDs to illustrate Pure Classical Pilates. And for the past several years, I have been both humbled and honored to teach in studios around the world, sharing the same practice that transformed my life.

If you are currently a teacher, I hope this book helps to strengthen your resolve in maintaining the integrity of Joseph Pilates' traditional method as you deepen commitment to your chosen path. And if you have deviated from the traditional method, perhaps this book work will lead you to consider returning to Pure Classical Pilates.

If you are a student, or if you are someone who has never studied Joseph Pilates' traditional method—perhaps not yet understanding its distinctiveness—I hope this book helps you achieve a more complete understanding and appreciation for Pure Classical Pilates.

> **Contrology helps prevent and fight disease by strengthening the body's immune system.**

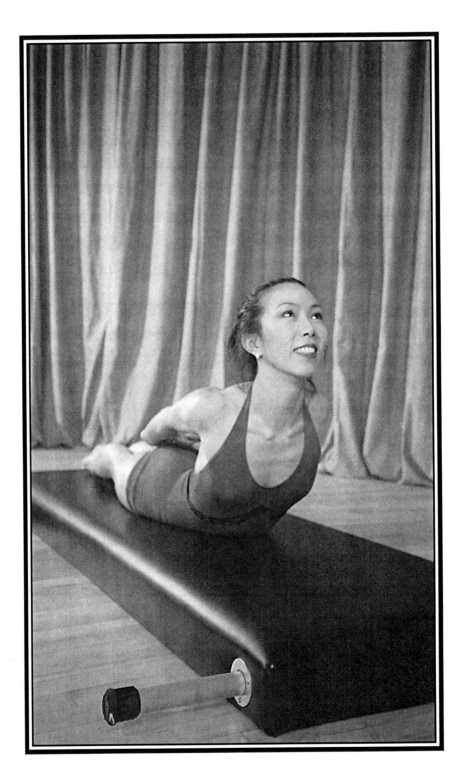

Chapter 2

Pure Classical Pilates
Inside & Out

Foundations and Beginning the Journey

Chapter Two

Foundations and Beginning the Journey

What makes Pure Classical Pilates compelling? What inspires devotion to Joseph Pilates' traditional method of body conditioning? What are some of the debates surrounding Joseph Pilates' system of training? These are just a few of the questions that may provoke interest in his traditional work.

Pure Classical Pilates addresses the wellness of the individual as a whole. Joseph Pilates designed his traditional system as a form of holistic movement to improve the mental alertness, carriage, coordination, responsiveness and precision of an individual's movement through strengthening of the core muscle groups. At a deeper level, the master's intention was to improve our chances of survival. Contrology helps prevent and fight disease by strengthening the body's immune system. He also created a unique and cohesive collection of exercises, which are sufficiently complex to study for a lifetime without inserting incompatible methodologies or movement techniques.

The historically accurate Pilates method is based upon an ordered sequence of exercises which is characterized by flowing movement, technical clarity, rhythm and dynamics. Within Joseph Pilates' traditional syllabus, there is a wide range of appropriate modifications designed to address various physical symptoms or limitations. While it may be tempting for some people, it is simply not necessary to include random simplifications, or insert aspects of other movement modalities into the traditional Pilates system. These intrusions are reductionist; ultimately, they detract from the complexity, intelligence, and cohesiveness of Joseph Pilates' traditional method.

Joseph Pilates' traditional work is both intriguing and beneficial because it is a *full body movement system,* utilizing full mental engagement or concentration. We *actively* stabilize certain muscle groups as other muscle groups are moving in a coordinated fashion. To achieve proper form and full muscular exertion, it is necessary to sustain complete mental concentration — or as much as possible — because we are always in motion, because we aim toward proper alignment, and because we initiate movement from the correct muscle groups, all simultaneously. The traditional method is a constellation of stable placement positions and mobility patterns. Pure Classical Pilates also has a wide range of movement vocabulary, yet the basic-intermediate levels are accessible to almost everyone.

Joseph Pilates first became interested in developing the system that he called Contrology (now simply called Pilates) to cope with health problems that he suffered as a child growing up in Germany in the late 1800s and early 1900s. He believed his system of Contrology (defined as the complete coordination of body, mind and spirit) increased the potential to gain a more responsive body; a more facile mind; and a fuller, more balanced life through his "corrective exercise" system.

It is important to remember that his traditional method is *a unique and indivisible system,* meaning there is intelligence and order to the exercises, each resonating with others and none working against others. In the traditional system, the progression of exercises form an epigenetic sequence:

each exercise — and each set of exercises — must build upon the proper placement, articulation, energy, flow and shape of the preceding exercise or set of exercises.

The traditional Pilates method is, first and foremost, a vigorous workout that challenges the mind and body in novel and creative ways. Joseph Pilates' distinguished protégé, Romana Kryzanowska, said there should be a sign over every studio entrance that reads, "Pilates is a workout!" And indeed, it is. Joseph Pilates drew greatly from his background in gymnastics and calisthenics. The intended energy-impetus and muscularity of his method should be strong, definitive and flowing, while taking into consideration a student's current aptitudes and limitations.

Joseph Pilates acknowledged that, while he did not invent Contrology, he famously coined the term. In *Return to Life Through Contrology*, he describes the athletic art and science of Contrology as the inclusion of diverse systems "...for regulating health and overcoming diseases...," which have been developed and practiced in different cultures throughout the centuries. He continued, "The traditional history of China affords us many instructive examples of the employment of various exercises to preserve and restore health" (p. 142).

In fact, Joseph Pilates specifically describes the mental and physical benefits of Kung Fu, originally developed in China. He further cites the training and healing arts developed in India, Greece and Rome. He makes it clear how "...the employment of Contrology for hygienic and medical purposes is by no means a new thing. In fact, it is older than any other means proposed for the same purpose. Contrology has been employed in every age" (p. 141).

Joseph Pilates' contribution, however, was to create his own unique rendering of body conditioning and, as he described it, "corrective exercise." His precise exercises, goals and qualities of movement were certainly based upon other disciplines practiced throughout the ages, but his qualitatively distinct system simultaneously aims toward improvement of mental, physical, and spiritual health.

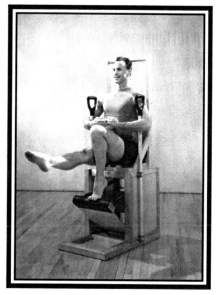

Today, Joseph Pilates' traditional, indivisible method of body conditioning is practiced and preserved by only a small percentage of instructors in the profession. In part, this is due to elevated educational standards of traditional teacher training programs, which are extremely comprehensive, especially in comparison to derivative and piecemeal training programs.

There are, however, other important factors that contribute to the limited number of traditionalists compared to instructors who teach derivative or hybrid versions of Pilates. For example, to train as a traditional instructor requires a significant commitment of time and finances, not to mention sincere devotion. In contrast, large international training corporations do not—and cannot—screen applicants for passion, talent or devotion, as this would require an interview and selection process for which most make no time. Besides, corporate business profit formulas are primarily based upon attracting high numbers of apprentices, with lower educational standards. *Quality is sacrificed for quantity.*

The attributes of passion, devotion and exceptional skill have been essential to Romana, Jay and Kathy Grant, as well as for many 2nd generation teacher trainers throughout the years. Even though traditional instructors continue to be a minority in the larger industry, Joseph Pilates' traditional method remains superior, as it is the *only* approach with a proven successful track record of creating health and well being since the early 1900s.

Applying knowledge gained in the traditional studio to our daily lives is beneficial in many ways. For example:

- When we walk down the street, we develop good carriage by lifting and lengthening up through the abdominals.

- When we throw a football or hit a tennis ball, we enjoy enhanced coordination and mental awareness by establishing movement in the center and directing effort through our limbs.

- When riding a bicycle or skiing down a mountain slope, we scoop the abdominals and allow relative suppleness in the torso and limbs.

- When we walk down a staircase, we negotiate improved relations with gravity by stimulating our abdominals inward and upward.

- When we are in the kitchen reaching into the refrigerator, cutting vegetables, washing dishes, lifting a heavy cooking pot or gently grasping a champagne glass, all the core muscles are working in concert to provide balance and grace.
- When rising from a seated position to a standing position, we motivate movement from the center to gain enhanced control and precision.

Whether picking up a young child, driving a car, running in a marathon, swimming in a lake, writing a letter, talking on the phone or engaging in countless other activities, developing the proper placement and movement patterns through Joseph Pilates' traditional method of Contrology is invaluable.

The 7 Cs of Pure Classical Pilates

In 1980, Philip Friedman and Gail Eisen published *The Pilates Method of Physical and Mental Conditioning*. This publication is perhaps the first resource to explicate the principles and technique of Contrology, after Joseph Pilates' own two books, *Your Health* (1934) and *Return to Life* (1945). And nearly three decades later, a majority of professionals still refer to Friedman and Eisen's description of six principles underlying Joseph Pilates' method of Contrology: Centering, Concentration, Control, Precision, Breathing, and Flowing Movement. Though Joseph Pilates himself did not originally define these six principles, they continue to be useful ideas for structuring our understanding of his traditional system of body conditioning, and have nevertheless stood the test of time and relevance.

Chapter Two

There is one more principle, though not outlined by Friedman and Eisen, to be considered: Cardiovascular Conditioning. As Romana and Jay would say, "Pilates is for the normal, healthy body." If someone is relatively healthy and symptom-free, a workout should be vigorous: the heart rate should sustain an optimum aerobic level for a particular period of time to gain cardiovascular benefits. Initially, students of Pilates will not experience this advantage, because the traditional method takes time to learn. Cardiovascular training occurs primarily at strong intermediate and advanced levels. One must first learn each exercise correctly; then, through practice and repetition, the exercises begin to flow, allowing the benefits of cardiovascular intensity and duration to be experienced.

The 7 Cs of Pure Classical Pilates:

- **Centering**: alignment, placement, positioning, emotional balance.

- **Concentration**: mental focus, short-term, long-term memory.

- **Control**: muscular stabilization, flexibility, breathing.

- **Correctness (Precision)**: placement, articulating shape.

- **Core Strength**: abdominal and spinal stabilization, carriage, power.

- **Cardiovascular Conditioning**: endurance, stamina.

- **Cadence**: flowing movement, rhythm, dynamics.

Concentration guides movement through Joseph Pilates' unified system of traditional exercises, thereby improving cardiovascular conditioning, coordination and mind-body awareness. As a result of consistent practice, one can expect significant gains in strength, stability, control, and flexibility, as all movement originates from what Joseph Pilates called the "girdle of strength" or Powerhouse region (abdomen, lower back, inner/outer thighs, gluteals). Students should expect to enjoy the following benefits:

- Lengthened muscles
- Improved posture
- Enhanced energy
- Increased mental concentration
- Prevention and healing of injuries
- An energizing workout

To apply the 7 Cs of Pure Classical Pilates in your workout is to honor the traditional method Joseph Pilates created. The tried-and-true arrangement of his traditional technique is a timeless concerto that sounds as good now as it did upon conception. Joseph Pilates' books and teachings, as well as his values communicated through traditional instructors, represent the sheet music he left behind. All we must do is use our skills to play the traditional composition and bring the movement to life—no rewriting, remixing or re-mastering required.

Joseph Pilates' Periodic Table of Elements:
Not Physical Therapy, Not Yoga, Not Dance

The traditional Pilates system can be understood as a Periodic Table of Elements by which our everyday physical movements, sports, performing arts or other body conditioning techniques are supported and enhanced. Conceived in this way, Joseph Pilates' traditional system of "corrective exercise" is a configuration of irreducible movements. As a Periodic Table of Elements, the system of Contrology is foundational in relation to various movement disciplines because it is a comprehensive system of core muscle stability and flexibility of the entire body that informs, guides and improves other activities.

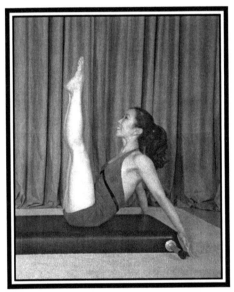

When people indiscriminately or systematically mix Pure Classical Pilates with other techniques such as yoga, dance and physical therapy, the integrated system of Pure Classical Pilates becomes diluted. Although physical therapy, yoga and dance are extremely valuable disciplines — each encompassing its own unique emphasis — when spliced together with traditional Pilates, they become incompatible foreign methodologies, working in conflict against Pure Classical Pilates.

Having made a point for retaining the distinctiveness of Joseph Pilates' traditional system does not negate certain benefits that come from training in another physical discipline. For example, when people have a background in gymnastics, sports or dance, they tend to possess general mental and physical skills that facilitate learning traditional Pilates — or a variety of other disciplines. These individuals can draw from their physical knowledge of coordination, balance, precision, stamina and the ability to translate a teacher's verbal instructions into specific movement. These students bring particular physical skills, intentions and nuances drawn from other techniques that can indeed contribute to learning and practicing traditional Pilates.

To the degree one's movement technique gained from gymnastics, sports, yoga or dance does not detract from Pure Classical Pilates technique, previous experience with other disciplines can facilitate gaining knowledge of Joseph Pilates' traditional method. Yet movement "styles" gained from other disciplines should remain implied so they do not detract from Pure Classical Pilates technique. If nuances or movement styles drawn from other disciplines become pronounced, or if people simply change Joseph Pilates' traditional exercise forms, the system of Contrology becomes distorted and less effective.

When people change traditional Pilates technique, the method is necessarily compromised; it cannot provide optimal core stability, flexible strength, alignment, coordination, responsiveness and mental skill that Joseph Pilates' classical method promises. All these beneficial qualities are a result of Joseph Pilates' Table of

Elements and, with consistent practice they become naturally engaged during our daily physical activities, whether we are walking down the street, driving a car, sitting down in a chair, playing sports or participating in various athletic arts.

Combining conflicting intentions, philosophies, and techniques of other movement disciplines into the traditional system, moreover, results in an attendant loss of integration, cohesiveness and effectiveness of the traditional Pilates method. While it is possible to slow or alter dynamics in the Pure Classical Pilates system to resemble yoga, or insert dance technique to make long aesthetic lines, these independently praiseworthy disciplines should not be incorporated into Pure Classical Pilates.

In order to understand how Pure Classical Pilates and other physical modalities may or may not work together, it will be illustrative to briefly examine them individually.

Pure Classical Pilates Is Not Physical Therapy

The activity of physical therapy relies upon evaluation and treatment of a patient's physical problem or injury, as well as the assessment of dysfunction that can lead to injury in the future. Physical therapy is a discipline of medical treatment, not a form of holistic body conditioning, a sport or athletic art form. Yet, physical therapy is especially worthwhile in the case of injury or atrophy, because it incorporates skilled manual techniques and exercises to re-establish normal mobility of joints and muscle strength and flexibility. Additionally, physical therapists instruct, educate and guide their patients to establish or re-establish normal movement patterns that have been lost due to compensatory mechanisms.

Physical therapy treatment does not contain elements of team strategy as in basketball, baseball or football; physical therapy does not contain elements of artistic expression as in ice skating, gymnastics or dance; physical therapy does not contain holistic body conditioning systems of movement like traditional Pilates or Gyrotonics. Instead, the emphasis of physical therapy remains on healing specific physical injuries, rather than strengthening the "communion" of body, mind and spirit alike. In contrast, Pure Classical Pilates aims to sustain and develop healthy, properly functioning aspects of one's entire mind-body. And, it is generally *after* a series of prescribed physical therapy rehabilitation treatments that traditional Pilates is considered excellent aftercare conditioning. Still, some physical therapists incorporate Pilates exercises in their treatment of patients to capitalize on its rehabilitative value.

Pure Classical Pilates Is Not Yoga

While yoga and traditional Pilates both aim toward developing a healthy connection between body, mind and spirit, the two disciplines originate from distinct pedagogical models. How each tradition achieves mind-body benefits differs greatly in both philosophy and methodology.

In my conversations with another instructor, it is clear there are many differences between yoga and Pilates. The two disciplines have two distinct descriptive languages, as well as divergent goals, intentions, historical sources and outcomes. Although we could debate particular subtleties of the following general differences, it is clear yoga and Pure Classical Pilates are distinct:

- Traditional Pilates is a system of body conditioning which is about 100 years old; yoga is a Hindu spiritual tradition over 5,000 years old with physical exercise being one component among many other spiritually oriented goals.

- Traditional Pilates seeks to improve our physical and mental capabilities for survival, strength and preparedness for action; yoga aims toward achieving divine enlightenment and God consciousness.

- Traditional Pilates encourages self-sufficiency and independence of the individual; yoga emphasizes a guru system of organization and connectedness.

- Traditional Pilates aims toward improving physical and mental conditioning so human beings can return to the natural movement and alertness of animals; yoga aims toward improving one's immune system and reducing stress.

- Traditional Pilates does not include meditation or chanting; yoga can include both meditation and chanting.

- Traditional Pilates emphasizes flowing movement and smooth transitions, often with gymnastic energy impetus; yoga most often holds specific physical poses for developing mental concentration and physical conditioning.

• Traditional Pilates includes specifically designed apparatus to lend support, alignment and structure to the body when practicing exercises; yoga does not conventionally include apparatus, yet some classes now have accessories.

• Traditional Pilates uses the breath to detoxify the body and expand the lungs, flushing the system with oxygen; yoga has a multiplicity of pranayamas, breath techniques, for glandular balance, immune system, altered states of consciousness, brain balancing, cooling, heating the nervous system.

• Traditional Pilates requires that our eyes remain open, thinking of how we establish movement from the "girdle of strength," how we direct energy with coordination and flowing movement between many exercises; yoga often has eyes closed, holding positions and thinking of God and transcendence.

• Traditional Pilates has over 500 exercises; yoga has at least 900 exercises.

• Traditional Pilates sources from Joseph Pilates' teachings, oral tradition, from his books and from the 1st generation of loyal instructors; yoga has teachers and scriptures, like the Vedas, Upanishads, Mahabharta, that describe the states of consciousness with the Supreme Dieties.

- Traditional Pilates is named after its founder; yoga, which means union with the infinite, has no individual founder.

- Traditional Pilates has few repetitions and flowing movement between exercises; yoga holds individual postures from a few minutes up to 30-60 minutes each, usually 1-5 minutes in beginner practice.

Although some of the postures of yoga may resemble those found in Pure Classical Pilates, it is in the emphasis and execution that one discovers their distinct differences.

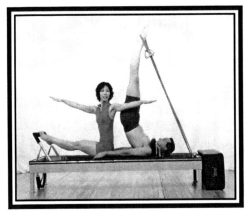

Yoga's goal is to *unite* the mind, body, and spirit; meanwhile, its style and emphasis can vary greatly. Pure Classical Pilates aims to *strengthen* the mind, body and spirit connection while consistently emphasizing control, precision and concentration. Understand, while a particular exercise may appear the same in both disciplines, looks may be deceiving!

Pure Classical Pilates teaches flat-back supine position in order to strengthen abdominals for maximum everyday functioning; yoga teaches neutral pelvis position, aiming toward equal distribution of force or balance. When comparing yoga poses to traditional Pilates exercises, the untrained eye may not be able to distinguish between:

(1) boat and Teaser, (2) plough and Roll Over, (3) bow and Rocking, (4) cobra and Swan Preparation, (5) chaturanga dandasana and Push Ups. But each exercise has a different intention, execution and is experienced far differently by the practitioner. Though they appear to resemble one another, these yoga poses and traditional Pilates exercises are actually quite different. Pure Classical Pilates will incorporate flowing movement within clearly defined purposes and shapes, while most forms of yoga will perform poses as static and steady.

Pure Classical Pilates Is Not Dance

In addition to physical therapy and yoga, some people have inserted aspects of dance technique into Pure Classical Pilates. As master teacher Kathy Grant clearly describes, there was no arabesque exercise in Joseph Pilates' traditional teachings. As with yoga and Pilates, there are nuanced similarities between dance and traditional Pilates. Yet, these similarities are limited. The energy-impetus and movement qualities of dance are distinct compared to Joseph Pilates' gymnastics-influenced method.

Dance technique has various movement styles with performance as the primary goal. Pure Classical Pilates technique has its own collection of elemental movements, but the purpose is for body conditioning, general health, as well as skilled applicability in everyday movement or athletic arts. Both folkloric and non-folkloric dance forms exhibit specifically choreographed patterns, as well as emotional or experiential themes. Oftentimes the aim of performance is to explicitly convey a story while producing attractive aesthetic lines. In contrast, Pure Classical Pilates is a non-performing educational activity where students learn body conditioning, although it secondarily emphasizes establishing clear aesthetic lines of the body. The traditional Pilates system, however, is not simply body conditioning. When it is properly practiced it can be an "emergent" athletic

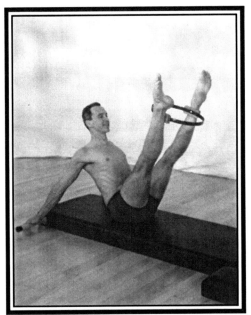

art form in ways that gymnastics and ice skating have become over the decades.

In my discussions with physical therapist and traditional instructor, Alycea Ungaro, she raised several excellent points regarding some of the differences between Pilates and dance. For decades, she says, consumers have mistakenly associated Pilates with dance and dancers. There are numerous interesting similarities between the two disciplines, but there are far too many stark contrasts to ever group the two practices together.

Consider the obvious. Dance is a visual art, a physical craft intended for entertainment purposes and driven by the experience of the viewing public. The shapes, movements and patterns exist only in so much as they are pleasing to the eye.

The physical conditioning which results from years of dance training is simply a byproduct of the work and by no means the intention.

By comparison, Pure Classical Pilates is intended for the practitioner only. Although it may indeed be awe-inspiring to watch a well-trained, traditional Pilates student work out on the Universal Reformer, the work is intended for the student only. There is no alternate "end-user" per se. The work begins and ends with the student.

Both traditional Pilates and dance employ similar strategies for goal setting and improving technique. The dancer strives for a higher leg, a loftier jump, and more exquisite pirouettes. But these improvements do little to benefit the anatomy of the dancer.

The perfection of such moves is superficial at best. As any dancer can attest, after years of honing their craft, the body is left much worse for the wear. Injuries and repetitive stresses plague the dance community long after the dancer has left the stage.

Quite the opposite, students of the traditional Pilates method can gain increasing physical benefit the longer they continue their training. Precision and excellence in the traditional Pilates modality yields a multitude of skills and abilities that enhance the quality of the student's life and well being. Traditional Pilates practitioners reportedly conduct their daily activities with far greater ease than those who deploy other exercise regimens.

Chapter Two

Perhaps the most striking difference between the two disciplines is the anatomical approach each technique employs. Historically, the dancer has focused on the limbs to the exclusion of the trunk. In fact, the dancer's trunk has been trained to be as mobile as possible in order to effect the fluid quality of movement required in the distal parts of the body. Think of it as a wave that undulates at the center and then reverberates out, away from the center.

In a completely conflicting approach, Pure Classical Pilates seeks to stabilize the trunk in order to mobilize the periphery. Operating from a stable support structure, traditional Pilates allows for the limbs to be free to move and thereby reduces the risk of injury. Perhaps seeing the error of its ways, the dance community has adopted a more traditional approach to trunk-strengthening protocols over this past decade, such as sit ups and the like.

It is interesting to note that, while dancers flock to traditional Pilates as corrective and rehabilitative exercise, the reverse is not true. Pure Classical Pilates students do not seek out dance as an additional training regimen. The relationship is not reciprocal.

One element binds the two methods together. The human body is meant to move through space. The resulting exuberance and sense of freedom that accompanies a well-executed workout is shared by Pure Classical Pilates and dance alike.

Suffice it to say, Pure Classical Pilates is not physical therapy; Pure Classical Pilates is not yoga; Pure Classical Pilates is not dance. Each discipline should be kept separate to retain its distinctive intentions and methodologies. Within the prescribed technical forms of Joseph Pilates' traditional method, we are simultaneously improving muscle length, strength, cardiovascular endurance and coordination in the entire body, as well as short-term and long-term memory skills. And while it may initially seem interesting to combine Pure Classical Pilates with yoga, physical therapy, or even dance — in actuality, this introduction of a contradictory style can work in opposition instead. Yes, there are similarities between Pure Classical Pilates and other forms of body conditioning; yet, these similarities exist because the human body is limited to certain combinations of flexion, extension and rotation.

Faithfulness to Technique

Technique is paramount at any level: basic, intermediate, advanced or super advanced. Interestingly enough, Joseph Pilates did not categorize his work into these four distinct technical levels the way we do today. He taught students within the framework of specific exercise orders and according to their individual needs, without regard to a specific technical "level." More important to Joseph Pilates was that his students get optimal mental and physical benefits from practicing his entire system based upon four necessary conditions: (1) flat-back supine position; (2) external hip/thigh rotation in most exercises; (3) calm quiet breathing; and, (4) flowing movement. These four necessary conditions are explored more in depth in Chapter 4.

Faithfulness to technique has additional connotations. For example, there are cultural differences between conventional gyms and the heritage of a traditional Pilates studio. To be sure, many useful activities take place in conventional gyms; yet, they are primarily in the business of serving the general public with a wide variety of physical exercise routines. Conventional gyms are more consumer-oriented in the sense that they frequently *adapt* to their clientele's preferences, and they teach various fitness fads when new trends come along.

In contrast, Pure Classical Pilates has a single tradition wherein *students adapt* to Joseph Pilates' traditional method — with his specifically designed traditional apparatus — in order to receive the greatest mental and physical benefits from their efforts. Of course, traditional instructors differentially apply and modify technique as necessary, depending upon the student's needs and symptoms, but we do not create new and different systems of exercise to accommodate any single individual. Nor do we insert foreign methodologies such as physical therapy, yoga or dance. The traditional method is comprehensive, and encompasses enough material for a lifetime of study and training, while still allowing appropriate modifications for particular individual needs. Adherence to technique preserves Joseph Pilates' traditional work and thereby preserves its effective mental and physical benefits.

The Educational Art of Teaching Traditional Pilates

Contrology, or the art of control coordinating body, mind and spirit, is grounded in an oral tradition of instructors communicating Joseph Pilates' values, movement qualities, technique and history to one another, and to their students. The relationship between instructor and student is paramount. Learning Pure Classical Pilates generally takes place in private lessons, duet lessons, trio lessons or small group Mat workouts with Wall Units (½ Cadillac apparatus). A traditional teacher provides verbal instruction, as well as hands-on physical guidance when appropriate.

In Joseph Pilates' original studio, students who became instructors worked for several years to become fully trained and to develop an adequate foundation of knowledge through extensive study, training and practice-teaching. According to Romana, Jay and Kathy, and many others who trained in his New York City studio, Joseph and Clara Pilates might begin by simply asking their more knowledgeable

Pure Classical Pilates has a single tradition wherein students adapt to Joseph Pilates' traditional method.

students to help someone with specific exercises. Gradually, a regular student whom Joseph and Clara trusted would be given more responsibility as a teacher-in-training. As the trainee grew to understand Joseph Pilates' method and how to instruct others, he or she would eventually be asked to teach entire lessons, integrating all studio apparatus.

It took several years to become fully acknowledged as an instructor by Joseph and Clara. They gave no formal examinations, nor did they require a specific number of training hours; yet, teachers-in-training did have to demonstrate consistency in their own practice and in their teaching at the studio. Joseph and Clara Pilates never organized a formal apprenticeship program, nor did they award graduation diplomas or certificates of completion.

During the 1960s, however, Kathy Grant and Lolita San Miguel were sponsored by the State University of New York in a time-limited career transition program that subsidized artists, actors and dancers to develop alternative vocations after their artistic careers had ended. Both Kathy and Lolita have certificates from the State University of New York that describe their completion of training under Joseph Pilates' supervision. These certificates are indeed impressive and they include a profound description of the traditional Pilates method. It may be worthwhile to note that neither Kathy nor Lolita was actually certified by Joseph Pilates himself; instead, they gained their certificates from the State University of New York. This point certainly does not diminish their studies with Joseph Pilates or their knowledge of the traditional method. Yet it seems relevant to ask why Joseph Pilates never formally certified students to become instructors.

Romana continued studying and teaching with Joseph and Clara Pilates for several decades. And it is important to acknowledge Romana's critical role of managing the original New York City studio after Joseph and Clara Pilates died. There is a sense in which Romana "saved" the traditional method by continuing the master's legacy in his New York City studio. During this same period, Kathy Grant also saved the method by teaching in New York City, then in New York

University's Dance Department. In Los Angeles, Jay Grimes also saved Joseph Pilates' traditional system by sharing his wealth of knowledge and experience over the decades.

Romana, Kathy and Jay focus their teaching in different ways because each person is unique. Kathy tends to emphasize improvement of stabilization and precise initiation of movement in pre-Pilates exercises, as well as basic and intermediate levels. Although, as a matter of course, Romana attends to these aspects of the work, she also emphasizes various other qualities, retaining the athletic artistry and practicing Joseph Pilates' entire range of movement vocabulary for those who are capable. Like Romana, Jay teaches the entire system of Contrology. When teaching workshops, he always includes an organized in-depth description of the philosophy of Joseph Pilates' work. Jay also emphasizes Joseph Pilates' traditional strong masculine approach and vigorous intensity. Of course an entire treatise could be devoted to illustrating similarities and differences of those who trained directly with Joseph and Clara Pilates, but it is beyond the scope of this book.

Learning the traditional Pilates system requires a minimum 600–1,000+ apprentice hours, plus regular private or duet lessons from a teacher trainer. There are also rigorous verbal, written and oral examinations included by the training studio. Conscientious instructors continue to study after graduation, because it takes years of training and teaching to become a proficient traditional teacher. After becoming a senior instructor, it is still a pleasure to study with knowledgeable colleagues and a traditional master instructor in order to stay on the right path.

It is simply impossible for students to adequately learn Pure Classical Pilates through self-study, partial training or watching DVDs. Of course, online certifications can never dispense the kind of knowledge and experience gained from traditional training. Neither can students learn the traditional method from overly detailed teacher-training manuals, which are produced and sold by large corporate certifying organizations.

Joseph Pilates' traditional method possesses great complexity and depth, and apprentices cannot learn the traditional work from simplistic and formulaic education. In order to become fully trained in Pure Classical Pilates, it is necessary to complete extensive education and teacher-training curricula in a traditional program and continue studying after graduation. There is no responsible shortcut and, depending upon the individual, it often takes five to ten years to become a knowledgeable instructor. In the meantime, we learn a great deal from just being students.

The Apparatus

As Joseph Pilates defined and ordered his body conditioning exercises, he also designed specific apparatus on which to practice them. The original apparatus designs are indispensable to correctly feel and practice both the intention and execution of his exercises/workouts.

He understood that we need to properly "process" the geometry and harmony of our movement to obtain optimal health benefits. In trusting the master, we should rely upon his judgment and retain the design, structure, feel and sound of each apparatus as Joseph Pilates created it.

Joseph Pilates' materials and designs are essential for preservation of the method. He created a variety of studio apparatus: The Universal Reformer, Cadillac, High Mat, Spine Corrector Barrel, High Barrel, Small Barrel, High Chair, Wunda Chair, Arm Chair, Guillotine Tower, Magic Circle, Tens-O-Meter, Magic Square and many other useful items. Over the decades Joseph Pilates experimented with various designs. One mechanism added resistance under water while stretching and bending the legs. He also patented a catapult apparatus. Was this a body conditioning apparatus or a weapon? Learning and teaching the traditional method absolutely requires Joseph Pilates' original designs.

In stark contrast to the traditional studio apparatus, several derivative equipment manufacturers alter Joseph Pilates' designs. As a result, they fundamentally degrade the athletic art and practice of Joseph Pilates' traditional method. It makes no difference whether the purpose of such alterations is to exhibit innovation, increase sales, or make the exercises easier — it is wrong. As a consequence of changing original apparatus designs, the remarkable mind-body benefits of Pure Classical Pilates can no longer be achieved. Since Joseph Pilates was the originator, his judgment should remain trusted and the apparatus should be true to his designs.

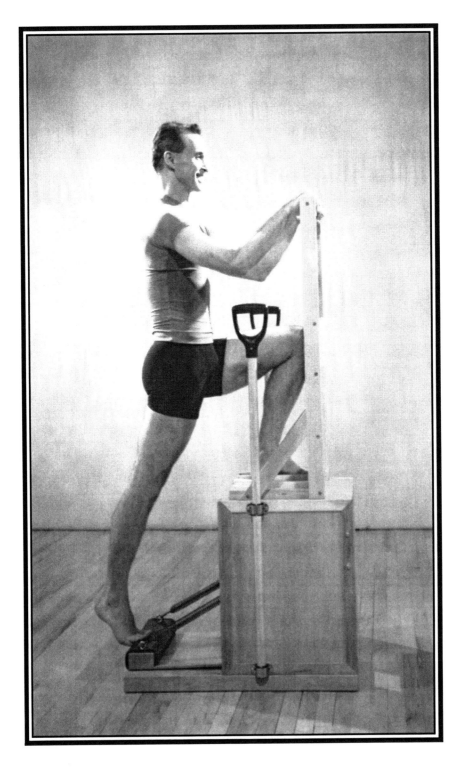

Chapter 3

Joseph Pilates:
The Making of the
Master and His Work

Chapter Three

Pilates and Paideia

Although commonplace biographical sketches of Joseph Pilates' life are widely circulated, these brief accounts have dubious origin. As yet, there seems to be no reliable historical account of his life with an accurate and documented chronology of events. Rather than simply restate these renditions of Joseph Pilates' life, we can safely say that his childhood schooling and young adult education in Germany was substantially influenced by Greek history, culture, physical fitness, athletics and aesthetics. It is not difficult to trace values and practices associated with European education to the influence and expansion of Hellenism—the spread of Greek culture and civilization—dating as far back as Alexander the Great during the 4th century B.C. (Jaeger, 1979). Throughout the centuries, educational systems deriving from Greek culture have included various aspects of liberal arts studies, architecture, law, family life, commerce, civic duty, moral integrity and good citizenship.

The concept of Paideia reflects Hellenistic cultural expressions and values with far-reaching significance. Many formulations in Joseph Pilates' writings parallel the tradition of Paideia: (1) achieving optimal health through body conditioning and sports; (2) proper ethical action in all matters; (3) becoming versed in liberal arts; (4) gaining the skills necessary to productively contribute to society; (5) excellence and beauty in life's endeavors; and (6) being a good citizen in the world. The concept of Paideia indeed has high aims for both the individual and society — and so does Joseph Pilates. As Werner Jaeger describes:

> It is impossible to avoid bringing in modern expressions like *civilization, culture, tradition, literature,* or *education.* But none of them really covers what the Greeks meant by paideia. Each of them is confined to one aspect of it: they cannot take in the same field as the Greek concept unless we employ them all together. Yet the very essence of scholarship and scholarly activity is based on the original unity of all these aspects — the unity which is expressed in the Greek word, not the diversity emphasized and completed by modern developments (*Paideia, The Ideals of Greek Culture,* p. v).

Joseph Pilates' education in Germany included the values of Greek culture and tradition, and he naturally modeled aspects of Contrology based upon these Greek ideals. It is not unreasonable, therefore, to consider that he implicitly incorporated concepts of Paideia into his system of body conditioning. Joseph Pilates clearly wrote about the virtues of Greek culture in his two books and endorsed their application to everyday living.

Paideia also reflects ancient definitions of privacy that are very different from today and which bear relevance to Joseph Pilates' method of Contrology. According to Georges Duby, Philippe Aries, and Paul Veyne, editors of *A History of Private Life,* concepts of privacy, subjectivity, and individuality during the Roman and Greek Empires were more closely associated with one's *civic* identity. Public life was more pronounced — and more synonymous — with every aspect of one's personal life, including thoughts, feelings and imaginings that we think of as private today. In the days of ancient Greeks and Romans, there was much less emphasis upon defining *inner* character, *inner* perception or one's "selfhood." In short, the difference between psyche and society was less distinct. One's inner self was more identified with public, commercial and political roles. Yet, over the centuries, definitions of selfhood and what it means to be an individual have expanded; therefore, today we have a greater divide between our private and our public life in modern-day society.

> **Joseph Pilates believed his method of mental and physical conditioning is integral to becoming a better citizen in the world.**

The concepts of Paideia and private life in Greek and Roman culture shed light on Joseph Pilates' perspective regarding one's health and well-being. He believed his method of body conditioning was not only a preventative medicine program to sustain and improve health through "corrective exercise," but also a system of mental and physical conditioning, integral toward becoming a better citizen in the world. Part of becoming a better citizen in the world includes making better moral choices, improving one's capacity to strive toward excellence, coping effectively with problems in everyday living, as well as cultivating beauty and identifying one's self more closely with social roles and functioning in the world.

Joseph Pilates' personality, as well as his approach to learning and teaching seemed to reflect ancient Greek and Roman definitions of private life. Although he was a tough boxer, circus performer, athlete, inventor, prison camp survivor and instructor who did not mince words, he was also a man of high ideals who cultivated individual accomplishment and the betterment of society through education. Joseph Pilates was a native German language speaker, and most accounts do not describe the master as talkative. Like the Greeks and Romans, however, he valued education; he was an avid reader and very knowledgeable about biomechanical principles and movement. He was a philosopher regarding physical health — or lack of it — and how it affects society as a whole. Joseph Pilates was also very articulate in his written communications to students and other professionals. He valued educating people about Contrology and how it can lead to optimal physical and mental functioning, as well as ideal aesthetics. Overall, Joseph Pilates wanted people to establish balance in their lives and to realize their full potential as good citizens in the world through cultivating proper values, work and action.

As the stories go, he was not interested in his students' private lives in the sense of asking about their feelings, relationships, job, family, vacations and so forth. In fact, many individuals who studied directly with Joseph Pilates consistently say there was very little or no socializing in his New York City studio. People simply did not engage in casual or convivial conversation. The point is that Joseph

Chapter Three

Pilates' character exemplified some of the high ideals of Greek and Roman civilization that he meticulously included in Contrology.

In a certain respect, Joseph and Clara Pilates considered their studio to be a center of preventative medicine, body conditioning and rehabilitation with professional decorum not dissimilar to a doctor's office, where promoting health and

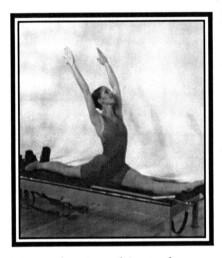

healing was all that mattered. It is widely known that Clara wore her professional nurse's uniform throughout the day when teaching students. Because Joseph Pilates was the originator and accomplished "doctor" of Contrology—in addition to being a self-taught professor of anatomy and biomechanics—his students were, to some degree, considered "patients" who practiced Contrology to sustain and improve their mental and physical health, thus becoming better citizens in the world. Again, Contrology helps prevent and fight disease by strengthening the body's immune system. Over the years, he was eager for his work to gain acceptance by physicians and the professional medical community. Despite writing two books, giving presentations to physicians and making short films about the effectiveness of Contrology, Joseph Pilates was unable to provoke interest in his method of "corrective exercise" from the community of medical professionals.

A Balancing Act Between the Mind and Body

Psyche was the Greek goddess of the soul and the wife of Eros, god of love. In our modern era, we tend to restrict conventional definitions of psyche to cognitive skills, learning, and memory function. Many professionals have moved away from early definitions of psyche, which include connotations associated with spirit and soul because they are not measurable or empirically verifiable. Of course important information can be learned from empirical inquiry, yet something is lost. Joseph Pilates, however, emphasized the importance of establishing balance between mind, body and spirit, both in his writings and while developing his system of conditioning.

Central to Joseph Pilates' modern version of Contrology are interactions between precise physical movement and mental functioning. He specifically trained students in mental conditioning by requiring memorization of sequential exercises, which both necessitate anticipation as well as coordination of energy, weight change, placement and creating specific shapes. Just as in any skilled physical activity or various performing arts, achieving precise physical movement in the traditional Pilates system develops practical mind-body coordination and responsiveness; it is very rewarding; yet, it can also be challenging and sometimes elusive.

Relations between precise physical movement and mental concentration reflect Joseph Pilates' deeper intentions. He believed practicing Contrology would improve cognitive skills in general, including aspects of memory, learning, judgment and concentration. He simply wanted us to have a more *responsive* body, a more facile mind, increased vitality, and a greater capacity to cope with problems in everyday living. In other words, practitioners would be trained and prepared for appropriate physical action and good judgment during everyday activities, as well as emergencies, should they arise.

In a sense, we create our own mental and physical balance through the way we subjectively assimilate the world. Although most of us have regular routines at work and at home, we also seek growth, novel experiences and various types of development that require us to achieve increasingly complex mental and emotional organization. Joseph Pilates speaks to this point in his book *Return to Life Through Contrology*:

> ...a Body freed from nervous tension and over-fatigue is the ideal shelter provided by nature for housing a well-balanced mind that is always fully capable of successfully meeting all the complex problems of modern living. Personal problems are clearly thought out and calmly met (p. 23).

To improve our short-term memory and ability to mentally focus, Pilates emphasized the practice of clearly defined, accurate, and precise physical movement for each exercise:

> ...beginning with the introductory lesson, each succeeding exercise should be mastered before proceeding progressively with the following exercises. Make a close study of each exercise and do not attempt

any other exercise until you first have mastered the current one and know its routine down to the last detail without any reference to the text. Be sure you have your entire body under complete mental control (p. 21).

During the early 1900s, Joseph Pilates countered prevailing educational precepts when he intentionally reduced the number of repetitions to practice for each exercise. He understood that practicing a single exercise too many times increased muscle fatigue and muscular imbalance.

...be sure never to repeat the selected exercise(s) more than the prescribed number of times since more harm will result than good by your unwittingly or intentionally disregarding this most important advice and direction...because this infraction creates muscular fatigue—a poison. There is really no need for tired muscles (p. 20).

By practicing fewer repetitions of each exercise, we improve our work in two fundamental areas: (1) quality of movement and (2) transitions between each exercise. Transitions *themselves* should be considered exercises because they require similar concentration and coordination.

Joseph Pilates believed activities of body and mind should be well balanced. He wrote, "...vitality itself is dependent on the absolute coordination of the body and mind." As mentioned earlier, he defined Contrology as "the complete coordination of body, mind and spirit." In his book

Chapter Three

Your Health, he asked, "What is balance of body and mind?" and then replied:

It is the conscious control of all muscular movements of the body. It is the correct utilization and application of the leverage principles afforded by the bones comprising the skeletal framework of the body. It is a complete knowledge of the mechanism of the body and a full understanding of the principles of equilibrium and gravity as applied to the movements of the body in motion, at rest and in sleep (p. 20).

Although we might infer what Joseph Pilates meant by "the body," he did not explicate concepts of mind or spirit in his writings. Because these subjects have been debated throughout the ages, he may have believed theorizing to be less effective than practicing his method of Contrology. He explains:

...the solution to our present-day health ills lies in recognizing the fact that normal development of both the body and mind is not possible by pitting the body against the mind, or vice versa. It is foolish to believe that one can perform effectively without working in concert with the other. Rather, by recognizing the mental functions of the mind and the physical limitations of the body, so that complete coordination between mind and the body may be achieved (*Your Health,* p. 18).

Joseph Pilates understood that mental life—if overemphasized at the expense of good physical health—can detract from people achieving overall balance and well-being. Sometimes a student would ask him, "What is this exercise good for?" According to Joseph Pilates' protégés, he simply replied, "It's good for the body." In the relative absence of analysis regarding mind-body relations by Joseph Pilates, we continue to train *experientially* with Pure Classical Pilates instructors, reflecting upon our teachers' comments, insights, values and stories sourcing from his New York City studio. Joseph Pilates may have presumed that we gain more complete experiential knowledge through direct engagement of the *entire* body. As a result, we have more capacity to understand how experiential activity implicitly translates into increased conceptual understanding of ourselves—and of others—as we become better citizens in the world.

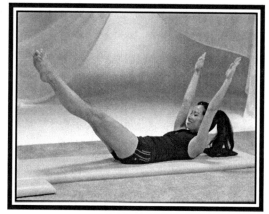

Joseph Pilates described that many cultures exhibited "an ever-increasing emphasis on mental training." Since educational systems and many professions primarily rely upon cognitive activities—sometimes at the expense of sufficient physical training or education—Joseph Pilates perceived most individuals as living in various states of disequilibrium. He believed Contrology could correct mental and physical imbalances caused by a cultural preoccupation with, even exaltation of, mental activity.

Joseph Pilates did not have a bias against conceptual learning or gaining knowledge. In fact, he was a strident seeker of knowledge to help improve the human condition. He simply observed that mental, physical and spiritual aspects of self fluctuate between states of balance and imbalance, and we can regularly work toward re-establishing balance through his system of Contrology. Joseph Pilates rightfully believed proper physical conditioning occasions optimal mental functioning. He wrote in *Return to Life Through Contrology*:

> The brain itself is actually a sort of natural telephone switchboard exchange incorporated in our bodies as a means of communication through the sympathetic nervous system to all our muscles. (p.54)

And he continues in the following paragraph:

> By reawakening thousands upon thousands of otherwise ordinarily dormant muscle cells, Contrology correspondingly reawakens thousands upon thousands of dormant brain cells, thus activating new areas and stimulating further the functioning of the mind (p. 54).

Yet his work goes far beyond awakening brain cells and stimulating the mind. Developed over many decades, Joseph Pilates created a coherent system of mental and physical conditioning that develops muscular balance, coordination, proper posture, breathing and skill that also improves aspects of cognitive functioning. Joseph Pilates believed it is absolutely essential to practice Contrology with precision in both mental intention and physical form. In *Return to Life Through Contrology*, he wrote:

> Concentrate on the correct movements each time you exercise, lest you do them improperly and thus lose all the vital benefits of their value. Correctly executed and mastered to the point of subconscious reaction, these exercises will reflect grace and balance in your routine activities. Contrology exercises build a sturdy body and sound mind capable of performing every daily task with ease and perfection. They also provide tremendous reserve of energy for sports, recreation and emergencies (p. 57).

Joseph Pilates thought it was important to refine awareness of our body and to intentionally train muscles in a cooperative manner to achieve uniform development with "minimum of effort and maximum pleasure." He also reasoned that subconscious coordination of our mind and body helps guide proper energy levels in daily activity and rest. Certain conscious abilities of mental and physical functioning are called upon to improve underlying (subconscious) aptitudes, which, in turn, advance these very same conscious abilities. This way, we can move toward or maintain optimal health and vitality.

Chapter Three

As our mind, body and spirit coordinate through the practice of Contrology, we can improve alertness and energy levels to sustain valuable relationships, work efficiently, attain reasonable goals and manage problems in everyday living. One purpose of Contrology is to help improve mental and physical *aptitude* in addition to practical skills. In turn, these aptitudes can be subconsciously available for balanced action and relaxation.

He continued to make the point that Contrology can provide "correct physical fitness with proper mental control." In *Return to Life Through Contrology*, he writes:

> As you progress in your self-instruction, you never have anything to unlearn. These exercises will actually become a part of your very self, securely stored away forever in your subconscious mind. Like learning how to ride a bicycle, how to swim, or how to drive an automobile, with Contrology one need never worry with respect to the possibility of your failing to use the right technique in these skills... (p. 62).

Although Joseph Pilates did not specifically define the subconscious, he did describe two other qualities of human experience that can be associated with interpretations of subconscious: instinctual movement and behavior, and spirituality.

He compared movement and behavior of animals, such as stretching, playing, hunting and resting, with human movement and behavior. He observed that various human cultural practices sometimes inhibit instinctual movement and, by extension, inhibit healthy living and mental functioning. One such practice popular at the time, and still in use by some people today, is the swaddling of infants.

During the 1800s and early 1900s, in particular, some parents swaddled their infants and growing children in cloth material, severely constricting movement of their arms and legs. The prevailing supposition was that children would continue their experience from the womb, and swaddling would help their legs stretch and grow straight. Joseph Pilates believed that infants, children and young adults should be allowed freedom of movement; then they should alternately practice some form of Contrology. As an observation in *Your Health*, Pilates noted that infants and children should have:

> ....the opportunity to freely obey their natural instinct, as evidenced by their desire for action, constantly turning around, grasping for and holding on to objects within their reach, stretching and bending their little bodies, creeping on the floor and playing in the sand or on the grass until their little muscles tire naturally, and then fall into a healthy sleep... (pp. 28-29).

Another common parental practice during Joseph Pilates' era was to "force" children to sit quietly in a chair in an upright position for extended periods of time. He went on to write:

> Proud (and unintentionally cruel) parents seriously interfere with and disrupt this natural course of bodily development by forcing their children to start walking or standing upright before their muscles have sufficiently developed properly to support their weight and before they have the mental capacity to control their equilibrium in movement. Normal children require no parental instruction or help in this direction…they will naturally keep on learning and trying until they are able, not only to stand in an upright position without falling, but also until they have acquired the ability to walk by themselves (p. 31).

A corollary of Joseph Pilates' understanding of the subconscious can be found by observing instinctual movement of animals. For example, he observed that cats achieve an "ideal rhythm of motion because they are constantly stretching and relaxing themselves, sharpening their claws, twisting, squirming, turning, climbing, wrestling, and fighting" (*Return to Life*, p. 16).

Although Joseph Pilates sustained his own conditioning through Contrology, as well as weight training and running, he actively discouraged overbuilding muscles from lifting weights, because the body becomes less limber and is slower to act or react. Rather, he believed that healthy muscle functioning, with proper proportions of strength and flexibility, is achieved by uniform development of muscles. He wanted people to gain suppleness and strength, as well as preparedness for action and appropriate response to emergencies. He wrote, "Contrology begins with mind control over muscles," so we engage critical thinking during specific exercise routines. One positive result of focusing one's attention to create precise movement is improved mental functioning. The proof is in the pudding; as a result of harnessing control of mind and body through Pure Classical Pilates, most people can simply become more physically

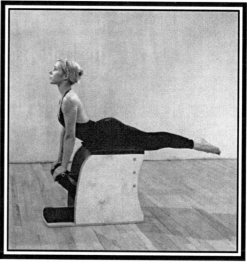

and mentally aware, responsive, balanced and symptom free.

The Spiritual Dimension of Joseph Pilates' Traditional Method

Without looking very far, we also find a long and rich history of writers who give considerable thought to connections between spirituality and the body. It will be fruitful to briefly explore a few historical texts that examine mind-body relations with consideration of spiritual concepts in order to illumine aspects of Joseph Pilates' traditional method.

Chapter Three

Although the discipline of Pure Classical Pilates is clearly distinct from the Indian spiritual science of yoga, we can understand both approaches in terms of being a physical ritual and a philosophy of mind. In the first volume of Sri Swami Sivananda's *Science of Yoga*, the unity or oneness of the body and the mind is the craft by which the yogi transcends emotional complication. The mental and physical exercise of yoga "...prepares the mind for the reception of

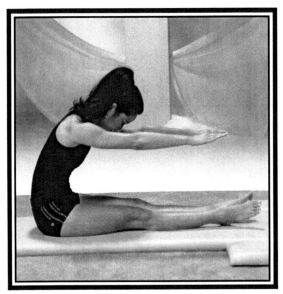

light or knowledge. It expands the heart and breaks all barriers that stand in the way of unity or oneness" (p. 7). According to the principles of yoga, all of an individual's actions, large or small, coalesce to form the tendencies which, in turn, develop character. The strength of someone's character, therefore, determines the strength of his or her will.

The strengthening of the will may take place over several reincarnations of the spirit through the actions of different bodies. The individual, according to Sivananda, is a free agent; the individual *wills* actions. Physical exertion through receptiveness to the Inner Witness that dwells in a man or woman can lead toward achieving oneness with the self.

In the *Tao Te Ching,* according to Lao Tzu, the approach to body and mind is one of willed separation. The goal of the soul in the *Tao Te Ching* is to separate from the body and bodily natures. The less dependent one becomes on the body, the less the mind and soul are troubled by the distractions of bodily life.

Striving for an ideal life of maximum separation from the body should yield freedom from mortal pains and sorrows and the assurance of being one with the universe. Lao Tzu identifies the soul as the life force in the universe; therefore, pure knowledge and reason are everlasting and know no death. Only the body can perish. The studied separation of mind from body allows no impact of bodily damage on the mind and, in turn, no impact of mental disorder on the body.

Another very early model of mind-body synthesis is offered in the teachings of Zen Buddhism. In the book *Zen Buddhism and Psychoanalysis* by D. T. Suzuki, Erich Fromm, and Richard De Martino, the authors set forth basic Buddhist mind-body theory. All parts of the body think, but, since the mind/head area and the other body areas have evolved in different ways and through different stages, the head and body do not communicate clearly with each other.

It is the Zen Buddhist belief that the limbs, abdomen and hands develop before the head. The legs and abdomen are closer to the earth and nature. The early development and closeness to nature attributed to these body parts lend them specific kinds of knowledge, which the mind and other parts of the body do not possess. Hence, the Buddhist notion that one "must not think with the head but with the abdomen, with the belly."

The *I Ching*, or *Book of Changes*, is perhaps the oldest preserved philosophical text, written some three thousand years ago. It is an oracle whose wisdom incorporates elements of mind-body harmony. The strength and clarity of the essence of being, as expressed in the *I Ching*, resonates throughout the history of philosophy:

> Contemplation of the divine meaning underlying the workings of the universe gives to the man who is called upon to influence others the means of producing like effects. This requires that power of inner concentration which religious contemplation develops in great men strong in faith. It enables them to apprehend the mysterious and divine laws of life, and by means of profoundest inner concentration, they give expression to these laws in their own persons. Thus a hidden spiritual power emanates from them, influencing and dominating others without their being aware of how it happens (p. 83).

Within Christianity, we can recall one of the most cited quotations from the New Testament: "...Or do you not know that your body is a temple of the Holy Spirit who is in you, whom you have from God, and that you are not your own?" (Corinthians 16:9). The New Testament of the Bible, though written by many of Jesus of Nazareth's disciples, contains several versions of his most important speeches. In these "sermons," he addressed several aspects of mind-body relations.

Jesus believed that, contrary to the religious doctrines of his time, sin can be committed in thought as well as in action: "...whosoever looketh on a woman to lust after her hath committed adultery with her already in his heart" (Matthew 5:28). He focused on the imperfection of the human mind and suggested that the mind can control the body in negative, as well as positive ways:

> Not that which goeth into the mouth defileth a man; but that which cometh out of the mouth, this defileth a man...those things which proceed out of the mouth come forth from the heart...out of the heart proceed evil thoughts, murders, adulteries, fornications, thefts, false witness, blasphemies: These are the things which defile a man: but to eat with unwashen hands defileth not a man (Matthew 15:11, 18–20).

In this passage, He characterized this imperfection of the mind as a lack of faith and a subsequent inability to rise above the earthly. Jesus insisted that this lack of faith explained His disciples' inability to heal the bodies of the sick.

Jesus did not locate all human fault in the mind, however. The mind can only negatively influence the body, because, as he declared to Peter, "the spirit indeed is willing, but the flesh is weak" (Matthew 26:41). Because of the weakness of the body, the mind can easily use the body as a vehicle for its own imperfect desires.

He recommended separating specific parts of the body that are serving as vehicles from the rest of the body in order to prevent the expression of evil thoughts through bodily actions: "If thy hand or thy foot offend thee: it is better for thee to enter into life halt or maimed,

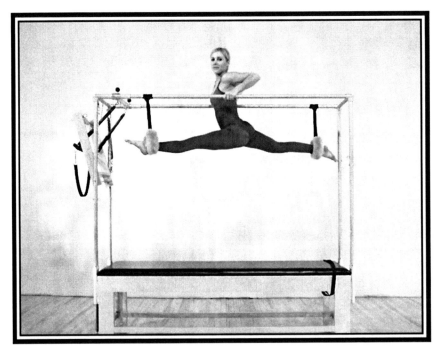

rather than having two hands or two feet to be cast into everlasting fire" (Matthew 18:8). Whether we interpret such a severance literally or figuratively, this passage suggests that the body may be fragmented, while the soul or mind is indivisible. The well-being of the soul may require bodily sacrifice if the body's weaknesses provide an opportunity for the mind to sin.

Even though Joseph Pilates included the word "spirit" in his often-cited definition of Contrology ("the complete coordination of body, mind and spirit"), he did not describe his understanding of it. Given that his native language was German, it is reasonable to assume that Joseph Pilates considered concepts of spirit too complex to adequately translate from German language concepts of spirit. According to all accounts, Joseph Pilates was not known to verbally express his ideas regarding spirit when teaching students in his studio, though he believed his system of Contrology to be both a physical ritual and a philosophy of health. In the absence of more specific information from Joseph Pilates himself, Contrology can be construed as a physical ritual that has varied and complex actions involving symbolic value. As a philosophy of health, Contrology is an educational system wherein participants gain increased physical health, emotional balance and mental skill that improve many aspects of their lives.

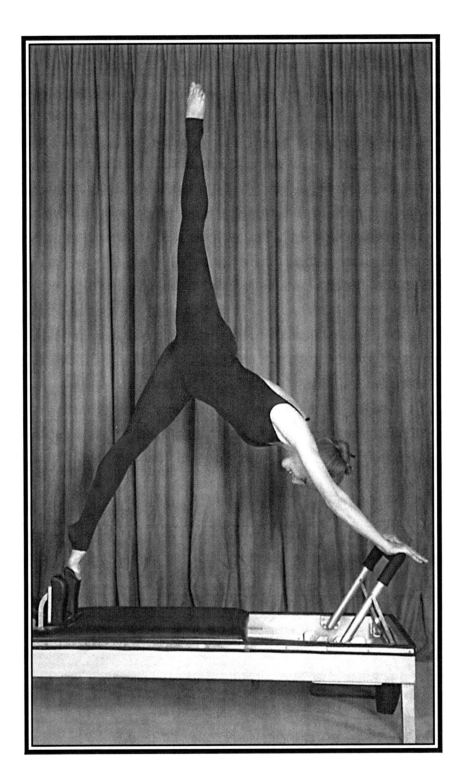

Chapter 4

Four Necessary Conditions of Joseph Pilates' Traditional Method

Chapter Four

Joseph Pilates insisted upon four necessary conditions to correctly practice his method of Contrology: (1) flat-back supine position; (2) external thigh rotation in most exercises, parallel position in many exercises; (3) calm, quiet breathing; and (4) flowing movement. This chapter illumines these four conditions and why Joseph Pilates insisted upon them.

The Flat-Back Position

When practicing and teaching the traditional method, all supine exercises (lying down, face up) are attempted with a flat back instead of a neutral-pelvis position. Joseph Pilates' reason for practicing flat-back position was for students to gain exact mental and physical awareness of abdominal action that produces increased stability, strength and articulation of the muscles governing the spine and trunk. As a result of this understanding, students can work toward decreasing symptomatic spinal "over-curvatures," as Joseph Pilates described. The flat-back position also helps to increase strength and improve muscular articulation that support optimal spinal placement and carriage, while moving into various other positions, shapes and motions such as upright kneeling, standing, walking, running, jumping, reaching, sitting, throwing, kicking and so forth.

Achieving a flat back when in supine position, however, is conditional to some degree, because certain body shapes physically preclude them from achieving a flat-back, horizontal position. At least, this can be the case at the beginning stages of learning the method. Due to one's anatomical and genetic framework, there are differences in the gluteal muscles, lumbar curvature and shape of the upper back that may create variations in flat-back position. There can also be structural differences as a result of someone's physical training. For example, swimmers tend to develop broader shoulders and upper backs; weight lifters and football players are known to have denser muscle mass; and long-distance runners tend to be slender.

For sure, there are many degrees of spinal curvature and many interpretations of a "flat back." So, when reading Joseph Pilates' books, *it is crucial to correctly interpret his phrasing*. When he uses the terms "spinal curves," "curvature of the spine," or simply "curvature," he is referring to medically diagnosable, significant curvatures (i.e. hyperkyphosis, hyperlordosis, scoliosis), that are outside the normal range and which produce problems associated with reduction in daily functioning and/or pain.

Although the general population has varying degrees of normal-range spinal curvature, Joseph Pilates was clearly not describing these individuals. He was focusing on maladaptive and pathologic spinal over-curvatures caused by poor posture evident in the vast majority of the "normal" population. Another point to consider—although it seems obvious—is this: when he described the importance of practicing Contrology exercises with a flat *back*, he did not mean practicing exercises with a flat *spine*. When Joseph Pilates instructed the use of a flat back in supine position, he was not suggesting we attempt to make our spinal column straight in this position or in any other position. In fact, this would not only be impossible, but undesirable as well, because we need normal-range spinal curvatures for standing, for balance, for movement, and for shock absorption. In *Return to Life Through Contrology*, he wrote:

> Because of poor posture, practically 95 percent of our population suffers from varying degrees of [abnormally pronounced] spinal curvature, not to mention more serious ailments. In a newly-born infant the back is flat because the spine is straight. Of course we all know that this is exactly as intended by nature, not only at birth but also throughout life. However, this ideal condition is rarely obtained in adult life. When the spine [has abnormally pronounced] curves, the entire body is thrown out of its natural alignment — off balance (pp. 58-59).

Everyone is born with a slightly curved spine. This arch, concave on the side facing the front of the body and convex on the back of the body, is necessary for the fetus to reside in the womb prior to birth. Once exposed to the effects of gravity, the spine will gradually bend and curve in response to the stresses of gravity and the increased use of muscles. For example, the neck will develop a C-shaped curve (front to back) as the baby learns to hold up his head against gravity. As the baby learns to pull herself to stand, the lumbar spine (low back) adapts to gravitational pull by developing a C-shaped curve as well. The thoracic spine (middle back), along with the sacrum (lowest part of the spine), are two segments that maintain a relatively forward curve, similar to that of the fetus in the womb.

With these points in mind, it is essential to understand that when Joseph Pilates refers to the spine as being straight, *he is not describing what is going on internally at the spine itself, but what we visualize externally about a person's body.* Through his obser-vation of the general population, Joseph Pilates realized that many people exhibited poor posture. He also noticed exaggerated

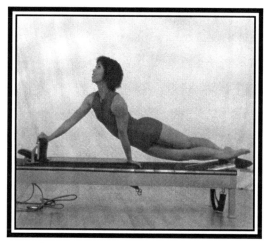

spinal curves from stooped shoulders to forward-jutting hips. He also correctly realized the relationship between these exaggerated curves and the rest of the body. When people are in a standing position, Joseph Pilates often observed their heads stooped forward and legs hyper-extended (locked beyond straight). Maintaining a posture of these exaggerated curves does not require much muscle control. Instead, this stance allows a person to be quite lazy. The body is simply standing and resting on its own joints and ligaments. While not problematic initially, this type of posture lays the foundation for maladaptive movement patterns, as well as a proclivity toward injury or reduced functioning.

The beauty of beginning exercises on a floor or Mat is that the firm surface along the back provides tactile cues to the sensory receptors of the back, offering constant feedback on alignment and palpable opportunities to self-correct. A student is instructed to *lengthen* the spine along the Mat or floor by pulling the pelvis away from the rib cage, slightly increasing distance between ribs and pelvic bone. This verbal description helps a student to activate the smaller back muscles, specifically the *multifidi* and *rotatores*. These underused muscles, which only cross two or three segments of the spine per piece, create a stabilizing effect on the spine, developing what we now term, "core strength."

Contrary to less-informed critics of Pure Classical Pilates, the flat-back supine position is not a static, contracted or "held" pelvic flexion, which some people inappropriately refer to as "tucked." Traditionalists are mindful of practicing and teaching directional energy with attendant muscular action, so that both the abdominal wall and the muscles in the back are equally and simultaneously lengthening. Students are encouraged to scoop and lengthen the abdominal area inward/upward toward the spine in order to activate a key core muscle, the deepest abdominal layer—the transverse abdominus.

According to physical therapist Aileen Chang, the transverse abdominus, along with the internal and external oblique muscles, are collectively the most functional anterior set of core muscles we have, as they take attachment onto the structure in our low back called the thoracolumbar fascia. This fascia serves as our body's own muscular corset; the stronger the muscles are that attach to it, the greater the stability of the spine. While the rectus abdominus, also known as the "six-pack" muscle, gets much of the attention in both fitness and fashion magazines, it is not a good indicator of spinal health or core strength.

In a healthy individual, the transverse abdominus activates immediately preceding movement of the limbs, as well as when the person is attempting to move on an unstable surface. In Pure Classical Pilates, The Hundred exercise is a great type of movement to activate and utilize the transverse

> **Flat-back position provides greater body position awareness to activate abdominals for use in lumbar stabilization during movement.**

abdominus, working as you lift your legs, head and shoulders off the Mat, then working it further by the pumping of the arms. The sensation of Joseph Pilates' Mat apparatus against the back provides a good indicator of whether good contact with the Mat is being maintained, or if the back is arching off.

Therefore, the purpose of working in flat-back supine position is to gain greater body position awareness, to activate and utilize the abdominals for their role in lumbar stabilization, and to facilitate internal muscular cuing of the segmental muscles to simultaneously increase spinal stability. All of these points are instrumental in allowing an individual to safely control his body as he moves through a remarkable number of whole body movements requiring combinations of flexion, extension, and rotation in various degrees.

Practicing Joseph Pilates' traditional method when we are walking, lifting, sitting, reaching, jumping, throwing, and carrying out various other everyday behaviors, will increase functional control of the spine and our abdominals to prevent injuries and efficiently achieve various physical movements with ease. Beyond simply achieving functional benefits, we gain "… natural grace, suppleness and skill that will be naturally reflected in the way you walk, the way you work, and play," as Joseph Pilates promises. In *Your Health*, he writes,

> …the normal spine should be straight to successfully function according to the laws of nature in general and the law of gravity in particular…the [abnormally pronounced] curve itself is especially dangerous to the vital organs and the body in general (p. 43).

Joseph Pilates explains the relationship between spinal posture and internal health—quite simply, a person who slouches will greatly reduce the space in the body for its internal organs to reside. In turn, this may impede the function and health of vital organs, such as the lungs, heart, kidneys and liver:

> Abdominal obesity and the dangerous effects of corpulence have their origin in the improper [abnormally pronounced] curvature of the spine. Proper carriage of spine is the only natural way to prevent against abdominal obesity, shortness of breath, asthma, high and low blood pressure and various forms of heart disease. It is safe to say that none of these ailments can be effectively treated until the [abnormally pronounced] curvatures of the spine have been corrected (pp. 44-45).

In "The Mat Exercises" section of *Return to Life Through Contrology*, Joseph Pilates clearly stated directions for properly practicing The Roll Up exercise: "Entire spine must touch Mat or floor" (p. 73). And Joseph Pilates' back is clearly flat in every photo of him demonstrating Mat exercises.

As previously mentioned, *The Pilates Method of Physical and Mental Conditioning* (1980) was perhaps the first and only manual describing the Pilates method after Joseph Pilates' own books. The authors, Philip Friedman and Gail Eisen, studied with Romana Kryzanowska while writing their book, long before the Pilates method became commercialized with various derivative interpretations.

Substantiating Joseph Pilates' directive that our backs should be flat in supine position, Friedman and Eisen write:

…press your back as flat as you can. Try to get all the air out from under it. Check by seeing if you can get your fingers under the small of your back. If you can, leave them there, and try to squash them between your back and the Mat. Feel the muscles work. Take your hand away without relaxing the muscles that are pressing your back toward the Mat. Press harder.

The authors furthermore depict a woman in several photos who is demonstrating with her entire lower back lengthened flat against the floor.

External Rotation as the Standard

The second necessary condition of Joseph Pilates' traditional method is external hip rotation or toe-out position. There are sound reasons why Pilates taught his students to position themselves in this manner.

There is importance in Joseph Pilates targeting the "normal healthy population" and trying to educate them about poor posture. As discussed, poor posture can be the result of poor abdominal muscle control, but it is also associated with femoral (hip/thigh) internal rotation, observed as a knee-in position. Why this occurs is straightforward: someone who neglects muscle control in the abdominal area in an attempt to maintain good posture is, likewise, going to neglect using the gluteal muscles to maintain good hip position. Additionally, once a group of muscles becomes underused and neglected, this group of muscles will naturally become *inhibited*. In this state, muscles "shut down," becoming weak and less toned. Over time, weakened muscles will hinder movement, impede physical adeptness, and likely succumb to injury.

According to Aileen Chang, when someone has poor posture with exaggerated spinal curves and forward-jutting hips, the psoas muscle, or hip flexor, becomes shortened and hypertonic. This change in physiology causes neural inhibition to the antagonistic group (the gluteal muscles), thereby helping to create conditions where the gluteals also become inhibited and cease to 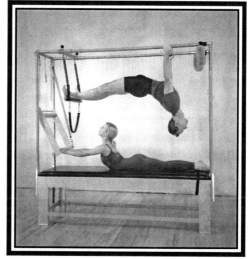 function adequately for our everyday movements, postures or specialized physical activities. Allowing this type of lazy posture also shortens the hamstrings and low-back extensor muscle, which, again, promotes inhibition to the gluteal muscles. Therefore, the gluteus is now able to hang out and be lazy, thinking that it does not need to do anything for the good of the person's body. This, however, is wrong. By pre-positioning the femurs into external rotation,

Joseph Pilates engaged the gluteal muscles, allowing them to "fire," thus assisting stability and propulsion of the skeleton in various movements.

Pre-positioning femurs in external rotation can activate the six deep external rotators and strengthen the inner thigh and buttocks muscles. These muscles are essential aspects of the "girdle of strength," as Joseph Pilates called the Powerhouse, and should not be neglected. External femoral rotation is also responsible for creating more stability when the body is standing upright. Moderate external leg rotation is the natural angle in which femurs extend from the hip sockets. It is no coincidence that the traditional "military stance" practiced by every military and civilian police force in the world is defined by external femoral rotation.

Since Joseph Pilates trained police forces in Germany and England, he understood that slight external leg rotation is the best position to support the torso or carry the body when standing or marching for long periods of time. Practicing external leg rotation is a necessary condition of improved stability, elevation, and locomotion. In addition, consider the standing position of gymnasts just before they run, jump and tumble in the open floor routine, or the position of gymnasts when they land a series of jumps — their legs are always slightly externally rotated, ensuring their stability and precise placement.

Joseph Pilates also included many exercises in a parallel leg position, because practicing both external rotation and parallel position *in proper ratios* encourages muscular balance.

In cases where a joint can move in two different directions, it is beneficial to strengthen muscles so that they develop relatively equal force potential. Remember that Joseph Pilates included more external rotation versus neutral parallel position because external rotators are generally smaller and weaker muscles; therefore, he intended for us to increase the strength of external rotators.

When practicing traditional Pilates exercises in parallel position, it is still necessary to activate hip external rotators, as this allows a carryover of muscle function in a more neutral hip position. By incorporating parallel leg postures into his exercise method, both the antagonist and agonist muscles of the hip and leg are required to work together to stabilize the lower extremity. This increase in gluteal strength will promote an increase in tone and, therefore, enhance utilization of the hip muscles in daily activities — and they will look better, too!

The "Ins and Outs" of Proper Breathing

The third necessary condition of Pure Classical Pilates is calm, quiet breathing. Respiration is a rather complex process that can be studied from several perspectives. You see, in addition to normal human breathing and its medical pathologies, respiration can be analyzed at the cellular level in plants and aquatic animals, as well as in fermentation of various foods. According to *Digestive System to the Skeleton* (Nagel, Frey, and Betz, 2007), "The main function of the respiratory system is to provide oxygen to cells and to remove carbon dioxide they produce" (p. 6). At a fundamental level, respiration is an exchange of gases that sustains the metabolism of a single cell, a group of cells or an entire organism. Stated more generally, in *Inner Focus, Outer Strength* (1996), Eric Franklin described breathing as "...a permanent and vital process that connects us intimately with the air that surrounds us" (p. 95).

In Pure Classical Pilates, we inhale and exhale calmly, slowly, and with ease, avoiding any tightening around the chest, or

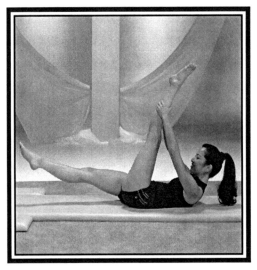

tension in the neck or the jaw. As the demand for more oxygen gradually increases during a traditional workout, breathing tempo may increase; yet, we continue to breathe deeply rather than to submit to a rapid, shallow breath. We calmly inhale through the nose, exhale through the nose or mouth—lips slightly parted—while increasing width and depth of our lungs. Abdominal muscles lengthen inward and fan upward into the back. This is true whether we are in flat-back supine position, flexion, extension, side bending, rotation or combinations thereof.

Jay Grimes says, "Breathe as if you are walking down the street." The point is to breathe "within" your breath to regulate a continuous flow of oxygen, while not becoming mentally distracted or physically distressed. Many non-traditional instructors overemphasize breathing, which can be problematic for students at any level. Traditional instructors, however, do not bother or distract their students by asking them to overemphasize breathing or practice foreign breathing techniques while practicing the traditional method. The key is to breathe naturally, calmly, deeply.

As a general guide, Joseph Pilates recommended inhaling during physical exertion and exhaling during physical release. As traditionalists, it is not our aim to create, or adhere to, a rigid formula wherein all movements must correspond to particular breathing patterns. Some individuals consider breath as a manifestation of spirit, and it is spirit that gives life to body, mind and movement. The point is to encourage effortless breathing, periodically emphasizing a strong inhale and a strong exhale as appropriate. Having said this, it is important to note the four exercises where strong breath is specific: The Hundred, Down Stretch, Snake and Twist.

Breathing quietly, rather than forcefully, during the exercises is important because it can carry over to daily life and function. While breathing intensely during a certain part of a movement may be helpful in aiding stability of the spine and activation of certain muscles, it is still necessary to keep the breath steady and calm. If a student can breathe normally through the physical exertion of the exercises, then when faced with strenuous events outside class that would cause most anyone to breathe a little faster and harder, the student can stay balanced in breath, balanced in life.

Breathing primarily involves external intercostal muscles and the diaphragm. During inspiration (inhaling), ribs elevate with activity from intercostal and intercondral muscles. As John B. West notes, "The most important muscle of inspiration is the diaphragm." West describes the diaphragm during inhalation:

> This consists of a thin, dome-shaped sheet of muscle that is inserted into the lower ribs. It is supplied by the phrenic nerves from cervical segments 3, 4, and 5. When it contracts, the abdominal contents are forced downward and forward, and the vertical dimension of the chest cavity is increased. In addition, the rib margins are lifted and moved out, causing an increase in the transverse diameter of the thorax (*Respiratory Physiology: The Essentials*, p. 79).

With respect to Pure Classical Pilates, Aileen Chang cites periodic confusion about the difference between activating the abdominal muscles to stabilize the trunk and the ability to breathe at the same time. In moving *inferiorly*, the volume of the rib cage increases, thus allowing the lungs to expand and fill with air. As we breathe out, the diaphragm rises back to its start position. At the same time the diaphragm moves downward, the ribs move to increase the volume of the trunk and decrease pressure within the thorax so that air may enter into the lungs. The ribs move in two ways. The first is like a "bucket handle," in that the ribs will move up and out (laterally) as we take a breath; in turn, this increases the side-to-side diameter of the thorax. The second is like a water pump movement, in which the lower ribs and sternum move forward and up, thus increasing the anterior-posterior (front to back) space of the thorax.

What this means is that during a Pilates workout, students are encouraged not to rely on the abdominals to assist breathing, as this is not their primary function. It is best to feel one's breath expanding the rib cage in its width and depth, while encouraging mobility of the trunk and spine as they facilitate good oxygenation.

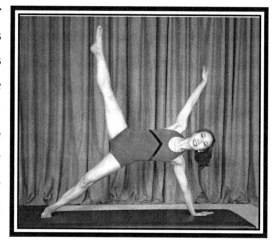

Short breaths provide a short supply of oxygen, while a deeper, slower breath transports more vital oxygen to lung alveoli. Because Joseph Pilates encouraged calm, quiet, deep inhalation and exhalation, he likely understood the biomechanical importance of breathing this way on a regular basis, and especially during a vigorous exercise workout.

In striking contrast to Pure Classical Pilates, there are varied breathing styles in derivative approaches: disciplined/undisciplined and conscious/unconscious. One example of inserting a foreign methodology into Joseph Pilates' traditional work is known as "percussive breathing."

Unfortunately, this type of breathing creates excessive muscular tension in the chest, neck and jaw, as well as significant mental distraction from coordinating flowing movement with strength and precision. In percussive breathing, the hasty tempo of respiration and intentional muscular contractions disrupt natural movement patterns and rhythms of Pure Classical Pilates.

Percussive breathing can be construed as a form of rapid shallow breathing (medically known as Tachypnea) without an underlying medical condition. Rapid shallow breathing can have several medical causes, including asthma, chronic obstructive pulmonary disease, chest pain, pneumonia and pulmonary embolism. Percussive breathing also resembles hyperventilation, which is ironically caused by anxiety or panic—not exactly our method's desired effect. This is not to say other forms of breathing are wrong or inappropriate for other activities, but these techniques should not be included in the traditional Pilates method. Again, when foreign methodologies are inserted into the traditional Pilates system, the technique becomes distorted and less effective.

To articulate this idea further, the term "over breathing" is drawn from music; yet, it is also used to describe symptoms associated with rapid shallow breathing, hyperventilation or dyspnea (shortness of breath). In the research article called *Breath Hold as a Determinant of Performance in Sports* (www.asthmacare.ie, 2008) "Over breathers experience greater levels of lactic acid, fatigue, chest constriction, breathlessness and poorer performance."

Some researchers have reported certain medical conditions could possibly combine with over breathing during physical exercise to actually cause asthma (Mayers & Rundell, 2006). This suggests that rapid breathing not only interferes with normal respiratory functioning, but also it can cause "exercise-induced asthma." This alone should be sufficient caution to those who feel creative and decide to change Joseph Pilates' traditional method.

In striking contrast to rapid shallow breathing, various relaxation and meditation techniques aim to slow respiration and heart rate levels. Although these breathing techniques are excellent for relaxation and meditation, they should *not* be incorporated into Pure Classical Pilates, because their purposes are very different. Relaxation/meditation breathing techniques purposely reduce energy to resting states, encourage convex expansion of abdominal muscle layers and facilitate greater movement of the diaphragm.

Joseph Pilates encouraged stabilization and lengthening of the abdominal muscle layers to provide a foundation for articulation and mobility in everyday movements, recreational activities or sports. Even in times when the body is relatively inactive, Joseph Pilates intended for us to have a responsive body and mind, always prepared for *action*. The body cannot be prepared for action or emergencies if we are hyperventilating or breathing in a slow meditative-relaxation state. To conclude, in Pure Classical Pilates, we breathe calmly through the width and depth of our lungs, while stabilizing and lengthening abdominal muscles inward and upward, whether we are in flat-back supine position, flexion, extension, rotation or combinations thereof. We are calm though ready for action if necessary or desired.

Fine Art of the Flow

The fourth necessary condition of Joseph Pilates' traditional method is flowing movement. Throughout the decades, Romana and Jay have devotedly worked to convey the heart and soul of Joseph Pilates' traditional method. As in Joseph Pilates' original studio, they strive to communicate the harmonious composition of all exercises. In this way, separate movements complement one another into an organized whole qualitatively beyond each particular exercise. Simply stretching and strengthening—in and of themselves—do not comprise the traditional method and they are *not* enough. In the traditional method, we not only practice creating shapes, but we articulate these shapes and refine these shapes.

With energy, coordination and focus, we aim toward creating a symphonic arrangement of all our movements. Our mind is the orchestra conductor, and our body is the symphony. Each exercise has its own tempo, its own "song," so to speak. It is essential to integrate our movement patterns with rhythmic patterns. In Pure Classical Pilates, we don't listen to music or watch television while working out, because the sounds would be at odds with our dynamics, inner rhythms and mental concentration. The teacher's instruction, tone of voice and associated images all help guide our changing rhythms and dynamics. Romana reminded her students, "Pilates is all movement. I can't correct you if you're not moving." Her point is that a teacher's verbal corrections cannot be properly integrated if the student is moving too slowly without enough rhythm or self-sustaining energy. The body cannot develop or exhibit proper coordination if movement dynamics are too slow.

Here it is important to understand that *coordination is a response to movement impetus*; therefore, we guide and control our movement only *after* we set the body in motion. If we control our movement too much, it feels and looks congested, stilted, and lifeless; if we do not sufficiently control our movement, it lacks 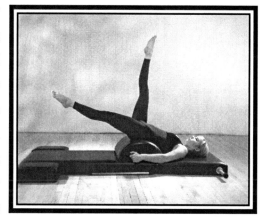 definition and integration in relation to other aspects of our body, as well as with other exercises. In Pure Classical Pilates, we first focus on functional benefits and then place emphasis upon transforming exercise into athletic artfulness or, as Romana would say, "Pilates is poetry in motion."

It is vital to distinguish between the athletic art of flowing movement and simply moving fast. Some derivative teacher-training programs push teachers and students into quick motion with less consideration of the person's individual aptitudes, coordination or skill level. Although these teacher-training programs describe their educational approach as having "flow," it is actually superficial speed that sacrifices essential aspects of proper movement quality, muscular action, precision, coordination and mental concentration.

Transitions between exercises are as important as exercises themselves. This point cannot be overstated. The dance happens between the pictures. Transitions reflect the subtler aspect of technique, because they require transferring our weight *between* exercises in an infinite variety of ways. Because of the nature of our body's muscle memory, consistent training is important: we must regularly re-learn how to properly transfer weight through various positions and balances. Learning how to smoothly change weight *between* exercises— while retaining stability, balance and control— is one source of feeling integration and coordination as we enjoy a good workout.

As Elizabeth Lowe Ahearn wrote, "All exercises and movements in Pilates, as well as transitions between exercises, are performed with fluidity or Flow of Movement. There is never any ballistic, static or jerky movement" (*The Pilates Method and Ballet Technique,* Journal of Dance Education, vol. 6, no. 3, p. 93, 2006).

Most often we don't notice transitions because our mental focus usually gravitates toward clearly defined "official" exercises. It is helpful to consider working aspects of exercise shapes within all transitions. And a workout with fine-tuned transitions holds twice the benefits. The athletic art of Pure

Classical Pilates requires *concealing* pedestrian transitions where our weight doesn't transfer smoothly. Minimizing extraneous or non-Pilates-related motion teaches both grace and efficiency throughout all movement, and is one of the secrets of athletic artfulness.

As a complement to transitions and a means of reducing non-Pilates motion, we have another goal of increasing literal and figurative space in the body. As we establish movement in the center, it is important to lengthen away from our center, creating more physical space between the joints and between each vertebra comprising the spinal column. This way, we counteract the effects of gravity pulling on our muscles and bones, contracting our entire body into increased density and less articulation. Creating more physical and imaginative space in the body can translate into achieving increased range of motion, improved stretching, and sensations associated with floating or soaring.

In a topic closely connected to efficient transitions, reducing irrelevant motion is crucial to developing any technique, sport or athletic performing art. There are infinitesimal points of balance within every range of movement. Readjustments or fidgeting interfere with balance during the range of movement. Every movement should have a purpose, and coordination is directly related to working *within* established movement patterns of the technique, the sport or athletic performing art.

It is also important to have awareness of what kind — and to what degree — we express various qualities of movement, such as suppleness, energy level, smoothness, sinewy strength, fluidity, sturdiness, luxuriance and so forth. These movement qualities arise from expression of one's values and imagination, and they direct one's movement choices. These qualities also affect the ways in which feeling influences form and how one's individuality brings movement alive in unique ways and in infinite variations.

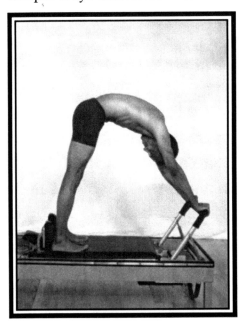

If properly executed, any simple exercise can become a source of physical and aesthetic pleasure for the demonstrator and observer. It is far superior for someone to practice a good basic workout with wonderful movement qualities, than to stumble through an intermediate or advanced level workout with inadequate training due to misplaced pride or ambition. Ego should never be the driving force behind one's level of practice. Quality of movement, placement and control should precede technical level. Only when an individual possesses an extraordinary combination of timing, coordination, precision, control and flowing movement can we consider describing the work as advanced or exhibiting technical virtuosity. Even then, there is always room for improvement.

It is also important to understand where — in the body — we *initiate* movement, how we *direct* energy that sustains movement, and how we *resolve* movement. With respect to initiating movement in a normal healthy asymptomatic adult, the transverse abdominus should first activate to help stabilize the trunk before guiding movement through the limbs and resolving movement. As an aside, when people have back pain, activation of transverse abdominus is delayed. This is why physical therapy aims to help these patients by first gaining transverse abdominals awareness and strength.

In keeping with Joseph Pilates' tradition, our goal is to create minimum effort with maximum flow. In this case, the word "minimum" means *optimum effort exertion*, no less and no more than necessary to create the best balance of harmony and intensity. If we invoke too much effort or overwork exercises, then energy coagulates in the muscles, leaving them strained and tense, thereby stifling the flowing movement. Conversely, if we summon too little energy, then the movement feels and looks lethargic, with decreased functional benefits. The paradox we must contend with is that *we get energy by giving energy*. On page 93 of her same article, Ahearn addresses optimum energy exertion in traditional Pilates wherein "…students must learn how to gauge their energy in order to achieve control and precision without a disjointed effect."

To highlight another aspect of the traditional method, we should sustain a good balance between internal awareness and external focus. Because Pure Classical Pilates is complex, practitioners tend to draw their attention and energy inward in an honest attempt to understand how to properly create shapes, while establishing coordinated combinations of stability and mobility. In this state, people become unnecessarily introverted in a quest to comprehend how various aspects of movement can combine to achieve the exactness of each exercise. Yet, when a student's attention is primarily drawn inward, it is not possible to create proper articulation of shapes or a desired expressive wholeness that is integral to Joseph Pilates' traditional method.

If we expend too much mental energy on comprehending technique, our work can become too internal and overly focused toward the inner workings of the body. This produces movement without "presence," without connection to others, and it diminishes important non-verbal communication between practitioners and observers in the studio—the very people who can learn by observing you working out. Certainly, it is necessary to understand how to execute exercises properly, but it is equally important to listen to the instructor's voice, translate corrections into movement, and nonverbally communicate a pleasant demeanor. It is more desirable to focus the right mental intention, which complements our movement as we coordinate both facial expression and visual focus.

Never should we attempt to hoard or hide positive energy during a workout! It is always best to radiate positive energy and share this uplifting sprit with other students, our teachers…and the world. When a student adds harmony and expressiveness to movement, this occasions a more complete and pleasing experience. It creates a shared realm wherein student and instructor can voyage together, appreciating the movement and getting a good workout while creating athletic artfulness. At a fundamental level, having an upbeat attitude makes the work more pleasurable and rewarding; subsequently, it invokes a central component of the tradition that Joseph and Clara Pilates developed over their lifetimes and so generously bequeathed to us.

To summarize, there are four necessary, though not sufficient, conditions of Pure Classical Pilates: (1) flat-back supine position; (2) femoral (hip/thigh) external rotation; (3) calm, quiet breathing; and (4) flowing movement. When you combine these four conditions with the unique qualities of each individual, Joseph Pilates understood that our everyday movements and athletic endeavors would reflect the practical strength, flexibility, balanced muscular skill, mental alertness, and energetic vitality that his traditional method provides.

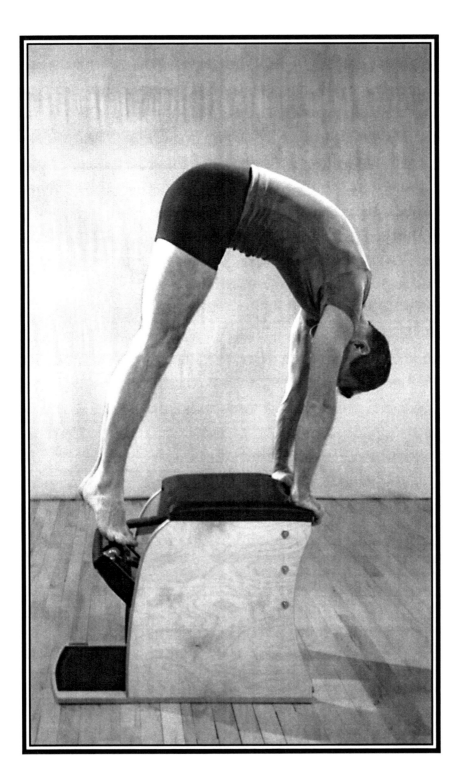

Chapter 5

The Body and Mind

The traditional exercise system developed by Joseph Pilates is as much a workout for the mind as it is for the body. As a psychologist, I have found it both natural and fascinating to consider how the two disciplines can overlap. I have developed a very simple self-reflection tool called Metaphors for Living, which is based on the 7 Cs of Pure Classical Pilates. This chapter begins with a brief description of Metaphors for Living and an invitation for readers to consider using it as they practice the traditional Pilates system.

The Traditional method and Life Lessons: Metaphors for Living

Because the work of Pure Classical Pilates is naturally energizing and intelligent, students often experience emotional growth and renewal in mind-body-spirit coordination as a result of consistent practice. Let us briefly take the benefits of Pure Classical Pilates to another level.

The *Metaphors for Living* concept is based upon principles of the traditional method, or the 7 Cs of Pure Classical Pilates as described in Chapter 1: Centering, Concentration, Control, Correctness, Core Strength, Cardiovascular Conditioning and Cadence. By applying these principles to our lives, we have the potential to deepen understanding of ourselves in a more complete way. I recommend periodically reflecting upon your workout experience to consider how these principles have a metaphorical significance in your life.

The purpose of this *Metaphors for Living* self-reflection tool is to increase one's insight as discovered through the traditional Pilates method. As a modest beginning, ask yourself these questions in relation to your work in the traditional method and create more questions of your own:

1. Am I applying the principle of *Centering* in my daily actions analogous to the ways I achieve centering during a workout?

2. Am I focusing my attention in my daily work and interactions in a manner that reflects the way I use *Concentration* in my lessons?

3. Am I developing aspects of mental and physical *Control* in my life similar to the ways I study Pure Classical Pilates?

4. In what ways am I demonstrating *Correctness* (precision) in my actions, speech and writing that are related to precise physical movement in Pilates?

5. Am I increasing emotional *Core Strength* in my life in the same ways that I achieve it in my workout?

6. How can I experience *Cadence* (flowing movement) as related to work, love, friendships and dealing with problems in everyday living?

7. Am I applying the *Cardiovascular Conditioning* of Pilates training to my life as far as endurance, stamina and emotional strength to achieve short-term and long-term goals?

Chapter Five

This *Metaphors for Living* exercise is a simple device for reflection that connects the principles of Pure Classical Pilates to our everyday lives. You can practice this yourself by considering the metaphorical significance of Pure Classical Pilates principles to your life, and developing your own plan for sustaining current constructive life changes and setting new goals for growth and fulfillment.

Pure Classical Pilates & Psychology: Similarities and Differences

Pure Classical Pilates and psychotherapy share a common interest: helping people increase self-knowledge and improve functioning in everyday living. Traditional instructors and psychologists are both healthcare professionals and teachers because, at deeper levels, they guide their students toward intellectual, emotional, physical and spiritual growth. Note the description of "student" (instead of "client" or "patient") for people who engage in psychotherapy because, in my view, psychologists are essentially teachers, and the activity of psychotherapy is primarily educational in nature.

Traditional instructors and psychologists realize that real growth is not isolated to just the physical or the psychological. And change in one area often leads to change in another. Similar to the work of psychologists, traditional instructors "journey" with their students—over the short term or long term—to help them overcome psychological obstacles and achieve general improvement toward becoming more complete human beings. Indeed, some obstacles are not physical but, rather, emotional, making it more clear why a traditional instructor can assist in psychological breakthroughs as well.

In contrast to the explicit activity of psychologists, traditional instructors *implicitly* work to help improve students' capacity to: (1) constructively cope with everyday problems; (2) develop insight and resilience to lessen inner conflict; (3) become more emotionally balanced and responsive; (4) gain more resourcefulness and vitality. Joseph Pilates' traditional technique, however, may offer an additional level of mind-body connectedness because of its focus on

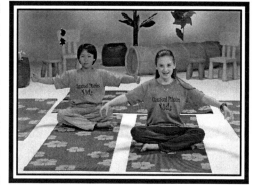

experiential self-examination, as students develop increasingly complex mental, emotional and physical skills to achieve progressively challenging movements.

As healthcare professionals, traditional instructors and psychologists set a good moral example as they impart values based on how they express themselves, which is not necessarily accomplished by disclosing personal information, but by sheer example. Actually, when healthcare professionals convey irrelevant or inappropriate information, this can impede progress by establishing a false sense of rapport and reducing important boundaries necessary for a student's growth and transformation. Irrelevant or overly private self-disclosure on the part of the instructor can be both inappropriate and counterproductive. Yet, sometimes, the instructor who shares information that is both relevant and insightful can actually forge a positive connection to facilitate a student's deeper understanding and growth. We are left with Romana's truism, "Use common sense!" as we carefully navigate through various communication choices in relation to working with each student.

As traditional instructors, we guide and support a student's strengths and aptitudes. Some students may have physical limitations, or they may have a normal range of emotional issues that are worthy of attention. For example, perhaps a student feels something is missing, not quite right, or a little out-of–balance in their lives. Maybe this person chose a career that is not satisfying, or perhaps is in a difficult marriage. In another case, a student might feel disheartened or lonely as a result of significant family conflicts. Another student might be experiencing depression and anxiety from going through a life change, such as relocation, working in new job, or dealing with the death of a loved one.

Even though a student may not directly communicate personal issues to gain direct guidance from a traditional instructor—as in conventional psychotherapy—there is a sense that instructors indirectly assist students to work through psychological issues *within* the parameters of Joseph Pilates' "corrective exercise" system. Toward this end, Pure Classical Pilates instructors support and "represent" the positive aspects of a student's psyche. We help maintain each student's healthy and resourceful impulses toward achieving movement skills, developing new psychological skills and attaining overall emotional health.

Similarly, a psychologist who practices talk therapy "represents" the healthy, creative and resourceful aspects of a client's personality. As Joseph Pilates said, "Physical fitness is the first requisite of happiness." His statement affirms the importance of having physical health in order to possess relative emotional balance leading toward growth and fulfillment.

Clearly, there are significant differences between Pure Classical Pilates and the practice of psychology. Unlike psychologists, traditional instructors are not assigned the role of diagnosing or treating emotional disturbance, revealing unconscious material, interpreting dreams, working through emotional blockages, 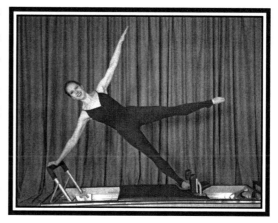 analyzing defenses mechanisms or transference. In talk therapy, the patient's goal is to explicitly *verbalize* feelings, analyze conflicts, as well as learn new, adaptive emotional-response patterns and coping skills.

Pure Classical Pilates instructors, on the other hand, help students *physicalize feeling into form.* In this way, *feeling becomes form* as it is transposed from mental intention into physical shapes. Then feeling guides our articulation and refinement of physical shapes. In the traditional Pilates method, we assist students in learning how intention initiates movement, how intention carries movement, and how intention resolves movement.

It is worth noting that there are physical manifestations of emotional difficulties. Poor posture, for example, may reflect a feeling of despair. Being "weak in the knees" can reflect anxiety or fear. Not "having a sure footing" suggests uncertainty. Being "hot under the collar" connotes anger. There is also a reciprocal relationship between physical and emotional states; for example, by improving posture, flexibility, strength, mental alertness and energy, one's mood can also be improved.

Another major difference between traditional instructors and psychologists is that Pilates teachers interpret psyche and body *in motion*. Since our body is to a large extent *who* we are, both mind and emotion are interpreted through movement. There is a sense that all emotion is "energy in motion." This is where Joseph Pilates' traditional system offers an additional level of mind-body connectedness— compared to formal psychological inquiry—because, in order to achieve progressively challenging movements, students need to practice *experiential* self-examination, training the mind along with the body.

Despite significant differences between the two disciplines, for illustrative purposes, there are relevant parallels to be drawn between Pure Classical Pilates and psychology. In varying degrees, and depending upon circumstances, both disciplines share the following structure and activities:

- Distinct teacher-student roles.

- A relationship that is both professional and personal.

- Regularly scheduled meetings to establish consistency.

- A professional who provides verbal interpretations leading to insight, understanding and growth.

- A professional who periodically identifies with students to "normalize" inner conflicts and obstacles.

- A professional who helps students develop a higher tolerance for frustration in a variety of situations.

- A professional who offers practical suggestions to create greater capacity for growth and fulfillment and balance in students' lives.

- A professional who supports and motivates students when inspiration and hope waiver, or when doubts undercut progress.

Traditional instructors establish rapport with students and attune themselves to their interactions of healthy and maladaptive psychophysiological trends. During the course of teaching, it is possible to observe numerous unconscious predispositions and personality traits by simply watching a student's movement. This is because movement is elemental and instinctual. The instructor gains significant psychological and emotional information intuitively, without reliance upon a student's verbal communication of feelings or ideas.

After observing various aspects of a student's mind and body interaction *in motion* during the course of several lessons, traditional instructors can explore uncertainties; provide appropriate and constructive feedback; develop options for achieving goals; and facilitate students to work through psychophysiological resistance. There is a sense that

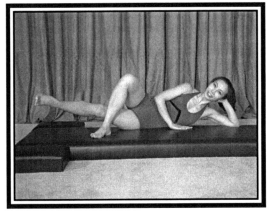

traditional instructors work *implicitly* as clinicians through the medium of Pure Classical Pilates. As instructors, the focus of study and treatment includes mind and body; yet, the primary focus involves the physical skills that actually originate from mental control, emotion and imagination.

Psychological Defense Trends Reflected in Pilates

Psychological defenses exist for a reason. They are practical and serve important functions for the individual and society. As a basic definition, psychological defenses are protection against inner disturbance, conflict or emotional pain—even though sometimes that pain can teach us something and avoiding it allows us to avoid important life lessons. Yet, employing psychological defenses repeatedly or continuously to guard against disturbing impulses/feelings can exact a high price insofar as they sap precious life energy and create problematic symptoms, including weariness, exhaustion, depression, irritability, anxiety, compulsions or anger.

During her extensive career as a psychoanalyst, the eminent writer and educator, Dr. Karen Horney (pronounced horn-eye), outlined three primary defense trends in response to unconscious "basic anxiety" of being helpless and alone in a potentially dangerous and hostile world. The first defense is *moving toward people*; the second is *moving against people*; and the third is *moving away from people*. Depending on disposition and experience, every individual tends to emphasize a single defense trend; yet, all three trends are simultaneously operating in varying degrees. It is important to understand the mind's defense mechanisms before understanding how these mechanisms can manifest in students, within the context of teaching Pure Classical Pilates.

The Compliant Solution

"Moving toward people" is characterized by helplessness and neediness. Some individuals are loving, warm and affectionate. Others may assume the role of a martyr. For people in this category, there will be general self-effacement, as well as forfeiting control and authority to others. This type believes in the power of love and the necessity of generosity and unselfishness. Due to their feelings of dependency, these individuals tend to display an unhealthy dose of humility. They will tend to be meek and unassertive and may actively strive not to be noticed or to make an impression.

Some, though, may unconsciously be more manipulative or controlling as they play the role of martyr. These individuals have, as Horney wrote, "…a marked need for affection and approval and an especial need for a 'partner' — that is, a friend, lover, husband or wife who is to fulfill all expectations of life and take responsibility for good and evil, his successful manipulation becoming the predominant task" (*Our Inner Conflicts*, p. 50).

The Expansive Solution

"Moving against people" is often characterized by inner hostility and great need for control. The expansive type will tend to be hard driving in whatever he or she is doing, whether in career, hobbies or even relaxation. These individuals have a need to excel and to be recognized. As such, they will surround themselves with others from whom they can receive affirmation. They tend to be wary and alert, always planning and looking ahead, and always on the scout for potential rivals. They tend to present a cool and unemotional façade, attempting to eliminate the complication of emotions from their persistent, competitive drive for achievement and success. They tend to believe that they are strong, honest, realistic and superior to others. Over time, their capacity for genuine friendship, love, empathy, and affection, is diminished. Individuals who emphasize expansive solutions to basic anxiety view other people as simply a means to an end.

The Detached Solution

"Moving away from people" is characterized by an exaggerated need for privacy and freedom. This resigned type uses isolation and distance—physical and emotional—for protection. This solitary type will probably avoid long-term obligations and relationships and will be particularly wary of the emotions and expectations that result from such entanglements. This type of person may also believe that spending excessive time in seclusion nurtures a creative genius. There exists an exaggerated need for independence, self-sufficiency, and authenticity. Furthermore, these individuals often consider themselves morally superior to others.

Defense Trends As Related To Teaching Pure Classical Pilates

Although there is an infinite number of subtle variations of defense trends within each individual, I will suggest just a few brief examples of how they relate to students in this context.

- A student who tends toward overdependence may abdicate locus of control and make the following assumption: *You, as the instructor, should work me out. It is your job to motivate me and keep me going. Take care of me and my needs so I may stay fit.*

- In contrast, a student moving toward detachment may suppose: *My body is a biomechanical machine, and*

I will achieve the best results if emotion does not enter into the workout. I will try what my instructor says, but I will retain my freedom to choose otherwise.

• And an actively aggressive student, who consistently initiates movement with "attack" and too much force may believe: *I must conquer this workout and dominate every exercise in order to feel I accomplished something good. I will master it, or it will master me. I'm frustrated, even angry, and I will channel my aggression into the workout. I should be good at everything I do.*

Links Between Psychology and Pure Classical Pilates

Perhaps it is not a coincidence that Joseph Pilates' Universal Reformer or Mat apparatus and the psychoanalyst's couch demand that students lie down. In the discipline of psychology, reclining in a horizontal position simply allows clients to listen to themselves without distraction, to relax, to travel back in time, and to freely associate thoughts and ideas. Analogously, in Pure Classical Pilates, students generally begin in flat-back, supine position to enable them to focus their attention inward, to listen and connect with their bodies, and to associate with the necessary muscles.

In flat-back, supine position, we do not have a localized gravity force pulling the weight of the head and torso downward into hip joints, knee joints, ankles joints and feet, as we do in vertical standing position. In the horizontal position, with the ground as a tactile cue, there is an opportunity to practice placement, alignment and muscular articulation with gravity's force being more equally distributed through the length of our body.

Flat-back supine position also provides the student with important tactile feedback from the Mat, Reformer, Cadillac or Barrels, because they support the back and, in some cases, the entire body. Supine position encourages psychological regression, which can actually facilitate psychological growth and progression. Psychoanalysts call this process "active regression in service of the ego" or ARISE. It is likely that Joseph Pilates intended for us to carefully consider our alignment, placement, length, energetic inten- 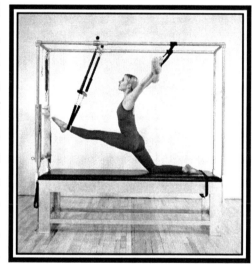 sity and muscular stabilization in a slightly regressive emotional state — yet more focused mental state — in order to prepare us for learning the complexity of his system. In the traditional method, complexity expands quickly as we progress from flat-back supine to sitting, to kneeling and standing positions with ever increasing movement vocabulary.

When a traditional instructor observes certain emotions communicated through a student's body (for example, disappointment, anxiety, anger or depression), it can be appropriate to suggest ways of working through these feelings. In other cases, students may manifest threads of frustration that unconsciously deflect from feeling unconscious self-criticism. Students may alternately come for help in actualizing their idealized self. In this case, if someone feels an inner drive to transform qualities or attributes into an idealized state, we can gradually help these individuals move from idealistic aspirations to self-acceptance. These students, with our guidance, may shift from working toward an impractical outcome and move toward appreciating the process and journey toward healing.

Again, our work as traditional instructors often includes assisting students in experiencing their true, authentic selves, helping them work with constructive trends toward growth and fulfillment. During this process, students may have to work through their own self-criticism, and even shame. Both psychologists and traditional instructors also assess the kind and degree to which students rely upon imaginary, unrealistic ways of perceiving themselves. The more a student identifies with exaggerated ego and pride, the more motivation there is to repress unconscious disturbance, thus staying put in an emotionally crippling, fantasy-constructed world. Attitudes and perceptions that comprise irrational or faulty beliefs are powerfully ingrained because they were created a long time ago during early childhood and young adulthood. They develop under the duress of basic anxiety and are used strategically to cope with the dissonance.

Another shared goal of traditional instructors and psychologists is to assist students in becoming aware of inner blockages toward growth and fulfillment. Over time, it is possible for students to gain understanding of how their faulty beliefs can impede overall health and well-being. As teachers, we begin working with students from the "outside", then move "inward," because we must focus on the conscious before we attempt to tackle the subconscious.

Individuals often demonstrate a degree of awareness of their problematic emotional conflicts. For example, some students do not feel good about themselves due to a lack of adequate physical conditioning or inadequate mental focus; as a result, they feel uncoordinated or unable to achieve certain exercises. After becoming more familiar with a particular student and establishing a good working rapport, traditional instructors gradually introduce stage-appropriate combinations of stability and instability to assist students' growth, both physically and emotionally.

Sometimes students seek a traditional instructor or psychologist when they are in a state of psychological deflation. Certain individuals have emotional or physical injuries and, as a result, may experience undercurrents of self-criticism, even failure. From the beginning, we need to be aware of the student's wounded pride and hurt. Yet, we should hold firm to the structure and definitions of our professional role. By doing so, traditional instructors and psychologists enable students to work at creating deep constructive personal change, while they grow beyond disturbed feelings, conflicts or problematic character trends.

As we assist students to increase their self-awareness, they begin working through and then resolving areas of inner struggle and conflict. Only then is it possible to develop higher levels of emotional-conceptual organization into a healthier equilibrium of selfhood. Sometimes, when a student is experiencing inner disturbance, there is increased motivation to constructively change behavior and problematic attitudes. This student is often more open and more able to reduce conflict and work towards improvement.

When students embark upon their first psychotherapy session or Pure Classical Pilates lesson, they sometimes want immediate relief from pain or a solution to an untenable situation. Both psychologists and instructors, however, help students reclaim themselves in a larger, more general, way. Although we attend to specific problems as professionals, we also acknowledge our students' positive attributes, their inherent abilities and natural endurance, in spite of all the difficulties. Naturally, we reinforce these strengths, while attending to specific, contextual and immediate concerns. This approach was directly paralleled by Joseph Pilates himself in his original New York City studio. When teaching students, first he reinforced a student's healthy physical aptitudes to strengthen the entire body, while simultaneously protecting the negative or injured part of the body from worsening symptoms. Then Joseph Pilates gave stage-appropriate attention in treating someone's particular injury or physical limitation.

Because most people have rivulets of mild self-criticism, one of our important roles is to help students practice self-compassion, appreciation and love. In order for more self-compassion to emerge, it is necessary for the person to become aware of disturbing or painful feelings. With respect to Pure Classical Pilates, obsessive feelings are sometimes associatively connected with compulsive movements, no matter how subtle or obvious. Students can gradually learn how they are emotionally *driven* — to one extent or another — by unconscious compulsions to assuage basic anxiety; how we are propelled to "live up to" unrealistic expectations of the idealized self; or how we strategize to avoid painful realities of the rejected self. Either explicitly in the psychologist's office or implicitly in the Pure Classical Pilates studio, helping students become aware of unconscious compulsive feelings is a useful task with beneficial results. Addressing this issue, George Weinberg writes:

> Often our purpose must be to help patients convert situational goals, which they present to us, into personal ones. Success is not to be equated with material comfort or even celebrity. The patient may pursue whatever worldly advantage pleases him, but what it will ultimately afford him is persona, and we must think in personal terms. A young man, not so bright, says he wants to become a congressman. 'What would that give you?' 'I'd be rich and famous.' 'What then?' 'I'd change the laws and give minority groups a chance, and they'd love me and appreciate me' (*The Heart of Psychotherapy*, p. 114).

As professionals, we help students understand that some goals can be unreasonable — or reasonable, depending upon the situation — but it is the unconscious strategies to achieve certain goals that comprise the sources of inner conflict. Weinberg says, "...we must think in terms of organic goals, of flesh-and-blood ones. They indicate a shorter and surer route to the persona's satisfactions than the one he has in mind" (p. 114). Notice Weinberg's comment describes "organic goals" as related to "flesh-and-blood ones." His point illustrates the intimate connection between our body and emotions.

Traditional instructors and psychologists should give students room to express themselves, either emotionally 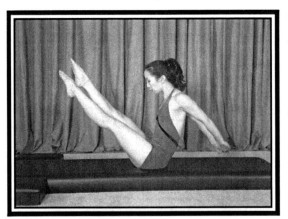 or physically. By allowing students more space, without interpretation or correction, they are in a better position to experience more self-compassion. Therefore they can recognize more of their positive aptitudes and strengths. This approach allows students psychological "opportunities" to gradually gain perspective and continue forward on the road of healing, change and positive growth.

Instructors should be aware of their profound influence, however, and exercise restraint when stepping outside the framework of their roles. A single comment or correction can have a lasting effect upon a student's life, like dropping a stone into the stillness of a High Sierra mountain lake: many ripples of meaning expand within the student's conscious and unconscious mind, as well as within her body.

Both psychologists and traditional instructors should avoid getting caught up in the internal-unconscious dramas of a student's life. Because the psychological complications and motivations of students are incredibly complex, it is wise to respect proper ethical standards in the working relationship. There should be a balance of perspective and compassion, as Weinberg describes:

Ultimately, there can be no replacement for showing we care. Not just the patient is precious but every human being, every center of human consciousness, is indispensable. There is nothing conditional about our patient's importance. We convey continually, 'You are the central figure. Your journey, which began even before you had power to reflect on it, is a magnificent one. It doesn't matter where you came from. In the chaos you made millions of decisions, learning, interpreting life as you saw it, furthering as best you could that single conscious being which is you. You were perhaps sidetracked and alone, or defeated yourself. Or you labored pointlessly in the wrong relationship, seemed almost buried alive. But your aspirations, like your heart, kept beating somewhere. Every stage of that journey was precious, and I admire that' (*The Heart of Psychotherapy*, p. 126).

Our work as traditional instructors strives toward assisting students with their strengths and struggles toward improved health. Yet, the work of sustaining and improving well-being can be periodically disillusioning. During the course of instruction, some emotional or physical symptoms begin to resolve, while others take center stage. In Karen Horney's view, some aspects of technique develop in relation to—and can source from—new and evolving understanding of an individual. Both psychotherapeutic technique and traditional Pilates instruction evolve from fluctuations in the kind and degree of someone's emotional difficulties and psychological makeup.

On a parallel track, Romana would sometimes say, "The method is right in front of you," when teaching a particular student—a particular body—meaning that we can discern deeper understanding of Joseph Pilates' traditional method *from the uniqueness of each individual.* So, there is a sense that instructors increase their own knowledge of Joseph Pilates' traditional system by drawing upon an individual's distinctive physical, emotional and mental characteristics.

Another purpose of both traditional instructors and psychologists is to help our students develop more inner freedom to open unconscious "doors" and discover varied aspects of themselves, gaining self-knowledge. In the case of psychotherapy, this process takes place through verbalization of feelings and examination of emotional or behavioral response patterns. In the case of traditional Pilates, this process happens through *physicalizing* feeling into form. As a result, both disciplines assist students to gain more patience, tolerance and an appreciation for their life's journey. It is less important for us to find out exactly what is behind those doors than for students to simply develop their own natural propensity toward self-reflection, growth and fulfillment.

The Pure Classical Pilates Studio: An Interpersonal Learning Lab

In light of our students' psychological predispositions and previous exercise histories, both students and teachers of Pure Classical Pilates find themselves in a laboratory of interpersonal and historical influences. The combination of these factors can make fertile ground for positive transformation. Our collaborative task as instructors and students is to work within the values and parameters of Joseph Pilates' traditional method as we grow and evolve together.

Traditional instructors themselves have unique predispositions, life experiences, personality trends and exercise histories. Even though we have extensive training and experience in Pure Classical Pilates, we periodically encounter unknowns and areas of uncertainty when teaching students with particular issues. Each lesson is a new exploration wherein we can understand our students more fully, realizing new information and knowledge. This is what keeps our work interesting.

At times, though, threads of uncertainty can produce anxiety within the instructor. In these situations, it can be useful for the instructor to observe and correlate personal sensations and body-memories when teaching a lesson, in order to understand students more fully, and continue providing the most effective educational service.

Sometimes an instructor will experience internal-physical responses to a student, even if they are scarcely perceptible. These body-based experiences can be an important source of

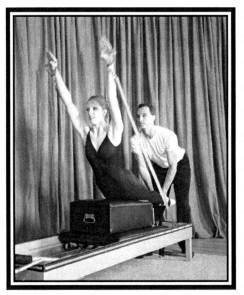

information from which instructors can deepen understanding of the student. During a lesson, for example, if the instructor is feeling tense or anxious, perhaps this particular emotion is unconsciously emanating from the student. The emotion, though unintentional, is communicated and then received by the instructor. The instructor's body is an instrument of nonverbal communication and, in effect, teachers can rely upon sensation and feeling to comprehend aspects of a student's unconscious psychodynamics before either the student or instructor consciously formulates such communication.

In contrast to body-based communication derived from the student, traditional instructors have their own sensation-memory experiences that arise independent of a student's nonverbal communication. For example, perhaps an instructor feels tired or weary during lessons with a particular student. The instructor may unconsciously project irritation or disappointment toward the student when the student lacks sufficient energy, not because the student has fallen short, but, rather, as a defense against his/her own conflicted feelings from another source. Depending upon the situation, such feelings can be acknowledged, contained or constructively channeled and not communicated during the teaching hour.

In this way, instructors can utilize indwelling, body-based feeling to gain awareness, then communicate new and useful information to the student. This educational approach can be a source of insight for the instructor, as well as a mechanism to help the student move toward wholeness, equilibrium, even transformation. It can be reassuring for instructors to know that our bodies have tacit knowledge that can be utilized to assist students when our conscious awareness is limited.

By placing more confidence in the unconscious wisdom of our body, which is based upon sensual and perceptual knowledge, instructors have the opportunity to be informed by, and learn from, body-derived intrapsychic events. After understanding the origins of certain feelings, perceptions and conflicts, the instructor will enjoy more openness and healthy adaptive functioning resulting from a new awareness of unconscious conflicts or blockages. Amongst the mental conditioning benefits gained through studying Pure Classical Pilates are improved:

- Overall energy level
- Self-acceptance and self-esteem
- Concentration and memory
- Optimism
- Coping with daily problems
- Sleep patterns
- Ability to relax
- Personal growth and fulfillment
- Overall image satisfaction
- Social involvement, friendships
- Overall emotional balance

Nonverbal Communication as Unconscious or Implied Meaning

It can be educational for traditional instructors to construe *implied meanings* from a student's physical movement, though not verbally expressed. During every lesson, there is a sense that a student's subjectivity strives to comprehend its own nature, its own activity, and its own purpose. As a result of Pure Classical Pilates, students tend toward creating higher, more complex unities of self-understanding that occasion fewer emotional blockages and less psychophysiological strain. Previously incomprehensible and varied psychic phenomena are brought into awareness, into more coherent and conscious meanings for the student, so that he/she may constructively utilize these aspects of self for growth and fulfillment.

Our quest is to *physically* formulate intention and feeling into action — into specific physical shapes — so we work through and express our emotions, becoming more complete human beings in the process. One of our indirect roles as a traditional instructor is to help students decipher implied unconscious meanings from within themselves because understanding these unconscious meanings assists self-articulation and self-realization. During every traditional Pilates lesson, an instructor takes into account various movements and gestures when attempting to understand and interpret a student's inner emotional

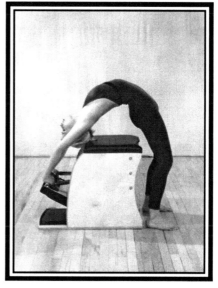

state and how his/her psyche is guiding feeling into form, guiding emotion into Pure Classical Pilates.

We also consider the student's quality of movement as he or she walks into the studio: the degree of tension or flaccidity in the body, alignment, posture, energy level, eye contact, range of hand and arm gestures. All of these qualities and movements convey important information about the student's mood, physical habits, conditioning, possible unconscious conflict and even character structure. Accomplished instructors are keen interpreters of psyche through the *physical* "expressive style" and idiosyncrasies of each person. Traditional protégés Romana, Jay and Kathy are brilliant at understanding *who* someone is by simply observing how he or she walks into the studio.

As students convey their skills, self-definitions, conflicts and strivings *through movement,* Pure Classical Pilates instructors can naturally "decode" both conscious and unconscious communication. Of course, instructors should not attempt to psycho-analyze students, as this is outside the scope of teaching. But traditional instructors do help students to become better at interpreting their implied meanings of self *through movement.* This includes helping students comprehend physical manifestations of mind, because we cannot rule out the effects of mental activity in any physical movement or symptom. In one respect, emotion can be interpreted as mind-body energy put into motion.

> **Physically formulating intention and feeling into action helps people become more complete human beings.**

Again, we should not attempt to turn Pure Classical Pilates into psychotherapy; yet, we can benefit from considering how memory, intention and purpose relate to particular movements, or an entire workout, as well as numerous workouts over an extended period of time.

As a student, you might periodically check in with yourself, making observations or asking questions. For example,

- "What was I feeling during this movement?"

- "When practicing this exercise, I remembered being with my family swimming in the sea when I was 10 years old; could there be significance to this memory?"

- "This exercise reminded me of playing basketball in high school. How do I feel about these memories?"

- "I was exhausted during the entire lesson. Could there be an emotional source contributing to my tiredness?"

- "I was frustrated at myself for not executing the proper timing of a certain exercise; what emotions and memories could be interfering with my timing?"

- "I had a dream about my instructor teaching me, and it was a pleasant experience. What could the significance of this dream be?"

These are just a few examples. I encourage students to ask their own questions, using their own words. The point is to explore relations between physical actions, memories, intentions and emotions for insight and growth. Working this way, the student has increased his reservoir of implied meanings from which he may draw significant insights and meanings. The instructor also increases available heuristic tools to understand and support a student's striving toward health and well-being.

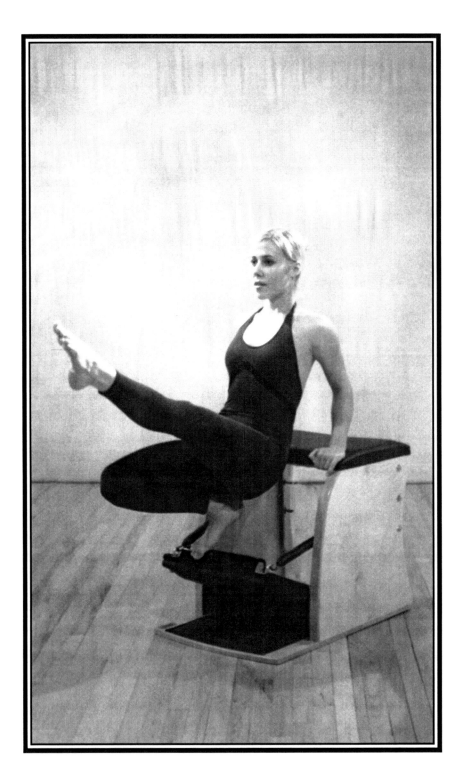

Chapter 6

Roadblocks to the Pure Classical Experience:

Small Business, Big Business and Rewriting Tradition

Chapter Six

Altering Pure Classical Pilates inevitably yields degraded strains, derivatives and hybrids of the traditional system. Whether someone changes specific exercises, the order of exercises, dynamics, or grafts an entire foreign methodology into Joseph Pilates' traditional method, his "body" of work becomes diluted. Watching Joseph Pilates' archival film footage, we see that he taught with strength, intensity and decisiveness. His traditional method of body conditioning is unlike varied distortions we see today: soft meditation-like Pilates, yoga-like Pilates, physical therapy-like Pilates, or large group classes using truncated Reformer-like machines lying legless on the floor. These examples are clearly mutations of Joseph Pilates' traditional method, and teachers of these approaches should neither describe nor characterize their derivative activity as Pilates. This chapter shall explain why.

The Great Debate:
Trust the Master or Mess with Perfection

During the course of his lifetime, Joseph Pilates taught thousands of students. If someone had the desire to become an instructor, he or she worked in the studio for an extended period of time, often up to three years. Apprenticeship was not formalized with a certain number of hours or a certificate of completion. Instead, students apprenticed by taking lessons, studying, listening, watching and practice teaching.

Joseph Pilates conveyed tacit and specific knowledge: tacit, in the sense of instructing students about his entire method;

specific, in that he taught particular exercises and themes of exercises for each individual's body. Sometimes Joseph Pilates created specific exercises and, on occasion, a specific apparatus for particular students, yet these exercises and apparatus had applicability to almost everyone. Another important aspect of teaching was assigning homework to students. The master regularly gave students exercises to practice between lessons so the movement patterns and muscle memory would become more intimately known in the body, and more beneficially understood.

> **Altering Pure Classical Pilates inevitably yields degraded strains, derivatives and hybrids of the traditional system.**

Over the last few decades, Joseph Pilates' traditional work has become misinterpreted, in part, because several students only learned the Pilates method through the lens of how he taught *their* individual bodies, *their* individual strengths, *their* individual limitations, and *their* individual idiosyncrasies. Therefore, these student-teachers learned particular, necessarily limited, aspects of the entire Contrology system. Unfortunately, when these individuals began training apprentices of their own, they only taught their limited interpretation of the entire method.

In contrast, Joseph Pilates taught both Romana and Jay the entire traditional method, as it should be taught to almost everyone. Joseph Pilates communicated his entire vision and technique to Romana and Jay, not only specific aspects of his method for individual physical conditions. Romana came to Joseph Pilates with a minor ankle problem she developed while dancing with New York City Ballet. Jay was never injured and he attributes his continued excellent physical health to studying the traditional method. As both Romana and Jay describe, teaching the "normal healthy body" with strength and vigor is the original foundation and continuing intention of Joseph Pilates. Yet, Joseph Pilates clearly understood the *secondary* value of rehabilitation.

Contrology was not originally created for rehabilitation, because it is meant to be a vigorous workout for mind and body. Though, given the assorted marketplace mutations of Joseph Pilates' traditional system, the occasional practitioner or general fitness consumer would never know it.

Misinterpretation of the traditional method can be attributed to the physical therapists, yoga practitioners, chiropractors, fitness instructors and self-styled industry personalities who attempt to create their own version of Joseph Pilates' work. They don't get it, and, therefore, neither do their students! Ineffectual attempts to change Joseph Pilates' traditional method lead to different types of degradation. Here are just a few:

- Making a disjointed collection of stabilization exercises, isolating aspects of the body and preventing vigorous muscular work with dynamics or flowing movement.
- Creating an amalgam of disparate movements without coordinated flow.

- Inserting rehabilitation exercises that are far removed from Joseph Pilates' original intentions and traditional system. While he paid some attention to rehabilitation and healing various common maladies in his original New York City studio, the primary aim of Joseph Pilates was to train relatively healthy bodies and relatively healthy minds.

In short, Pure Classical Pilates intends to sustain and increase *current* physical and mental health. This point is central to Joseph Pilates' philosophy. And though Joseph Pilates indeed taught his method to people who had injuries, the traditional system does not limit its focus to rehabilitation. Sadly, most training centers in the world have lost essential elements of Joseph Pilates' practice and vision. Most teacher trainers have never learned the foundations and technique as a coherent system, 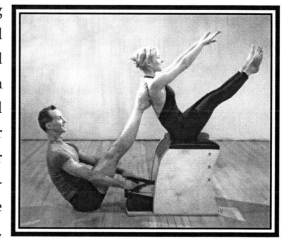 and others simply change the traditional method for expediency and profit.

Deterioration of Pure Classical Pilates stems from ignorance or, dare I say, arrogance. Without seriously considering the potential harm, teachers often haphazardly splice aspects of physical therapy, yoga, chiropractic placement, dance and other disciplines into Joseph Pilates' traditional method. Or, worse, many people simply create new exercises however they please. In either case, changing the traditional system impairs its benefits.

Some derivative approaches stem from fitness industry professionals and personal trainers who might take *a single lesson*, perhaps a few lessons or a weekend certification course in order to incorporate Pilates into their aerobics, weight-lifting, or circuit training classes. This unconscionable approach dilutes the effectiveness of Joseph Pilates' traditional method—in addition to unethically offering a service outside the personal trainer's scope of expertise. Having made this point, however, there can certainly be value in loyal traditional instructors who have training in other disciplines. One such instructor, Alycea Ungaro, who is also a licensed physical therapist, shared one day, "I teach the traditional method through a physical therapist's eyes." Her statement demonstrates how modern scientific knowledge of biomechanical principles and rehabilitation can coexist with, and indeed confirm the efficacy of, Joseph Pilates' traditional principles and technique.

Traditionalists don't compromise Joseph Pilates' principles and values for trendy, marketable counterfeits of the pure method in the ways mentioned above. Nor do traditionalists incorporate stretch bands, balls, rollers and other props that Joseph Pilates did not employ. Traditionalists only use Joseph Pilates' accessory apparatus, such as the Magic Circle, Toe Corrector, Foot Corrector, Magic Square (Neck Stretcher), Tens-O-Meter, Bean Bag Roll-Up Device, Breath-A-Cizor and so forth.

The Great Decline:
Derivative Styles of the Traditional method

Before characterizing derivative distortions of traditional technique, let the record state, we traditionalists are not an exclusive group: *In fact, you are welcome to join us. We invite you to study the traditional method and become one of us!*

Many traditionalists are forging a new era of open communication and enthusiasm for sharing knowledge. For example, in 2007, there was a gathering of experienced traditional instructors where participants from all backgrounds were welcome. More traditionalists produced similar events in Dallas and Chicago during 2008-2009. Dana Santi is organizing a Traditional Pilates Intensive near Chicago in April 2009. These events include traditional instructors and they are open to the public. By all reports, participants from every background were pleased with the hospitality and collegial atmosphere of the first two conferences.

Over time, I have gladly noticed increasing numbers of instructors trained by non-traditional schools gravitating toward traditional ways of teaching and practicing Joseph Pilates' pure method. Scores of very skilled, positive traditional teachers are actively teaching Joseph Pilates' traditional system and forging new connections with various professionals from every background. Traditionalists understand that the highest mental and physical benefits come from Joseph Pilates' complete and indivisible system as he originally created it. In spite of our best efforts to preserve his traditional work, unfortunately, there are people who attempt to "re-invent" the wheel. This is impossible without damaging Joseph Pilates' intentions, design and practice of Contrology.

Actually, derivative approaches of Joseph Pilates' traditional method were developing long before he died in 1967, as some instructors relocated away from New York City and started their own studios and training centers, primarily in the western United States. Although trained directly by Joseph Pilates, some of these individuals purposely altered the traditional method, supposing certain changes were useful or necessary. Perhaps these teachers had worthwhile ideas, yet changing the traditional method is by definition, derivative, which inevitably reduces the comprehensiveness and effectiveness of Contrology.

I have taught many people who were trained in derivative versions of Joseph Pilates' traditional method. In contrast to the high ideals and teaching practices defined by the master, these instructors and students exhibit skills that are less than complete regarding mental concentration, precision, flowing movement, strength, coordination or smooth transitions. Lack of good technical training and degradation of the method, however, are not the student's fault. There are innumerable students who are wonderful people with good intentions and sound abilities, yet they have simply found the wrong training center or studio. This is indeed regrettable, yet it happens all too frequently. These people do not even know the difference between Pure Classical Pilates and derivative approaches.

Mutations of the traditional method have slowly, insidiously spread for decades. In fact, some of Joseph Pilates' own students would publicly say they were teaching *their own version* of Joseph Pilates' original intentions. Yet, it is with false presumption that they set out to "improve" Joseph Pilates' unique creation. They did not sufficiently analyze the depths of Joseph Pilates' philosophy as related to his body conditioning technique and effectiveness for students. Their understanding of the traditional method was necessarily limited and their work deviates from Joseph Pilates' theory and practice.

Admittedly, there is truth to the slightly sarcastic comment made by one extraordinary instructor, "Even bad Pilates can be good for you." This point is that simply walking down the street can be mildly beneficial for the body, as well. Most safe movement can be relatively good for you no matter how undisciplined, unsystematic, piecemeal or generic. Yet, these characteristics have nothing to do with Joseph Pilates' traditional method, which is based upon systematic technique that results in improved mental and physical health.

Since the early 1990s, the Pilates business has expanded and grown in popularity. From approximately 1990-2000, studio owners and teacher-training programs were prohibited from publicly using the word "Pilates" in any business name because of trademark restrictions. In October 2000, when a U.S. Federal District Court ruled the word "Pilates" could not be a trademark-protected name, mutations and derivatives spread like wildfire. Thousands of instructors and business people around the world created their own teacher-training programs and recorded their own DVDs to increase brand name recognition; to build their reputations; and to increase financial success in the new burgeoning business of Pilates. The new business of Pilates was quickly becoming a mainstream activity in the growing health and fitness industry.

The post-2000 marketplace explosion of commercialized Pilates has been joined by derivative equipment manufacturers eager to sell infinite quantities of equipment, adapting traditional apparatus to a cacophony of business practices and consumer preferences, thus making Pilates more palatable for increasing numbers of consumers. Scores of teachers, training organizations and manufacturers have purposely digressed from Joseph Pilates' traditional work in exchange for increasing equipment sales and filling apprenticeship slots as they establish relative power, prestige and privilege in the brand new *Pilates industry.* Although we can only speculate, one reason why many small independent studios, self-styled industry personalities and international corporations change the traditional method can be described as technique alteration for profit generation.

Another reason people change the traditional method is because they truly believe Joseph Pilates' traditional method can be improved. Yet, as previously mentioned, their efforts are piecemeal and compromised by ignorance, even self-deception. Many corporate, teacher-training organizations fundamentally alter traditional technique and lower training standards in order to cast the widest possible net, and to enroll large numbers of apprentices and students into their global network of studios.

The purpose of lowering technique and training standards is to make the method more digestible and more accessible to the public. These changes can certainly make Pilates more palatable to apprentices and the public, but they disregard Joseph Pilates' rigorous standards of education and do not utilize each person's full aptitude, skill, disposition, desire and commitment. Larger scale corporate teacher-training programs do not set program standards at the highest level for two primary reasons: (1) corporate leadership often does not have the in-depth knowledge of Joseph Pilates' traditional method; and (2) setting reasonably 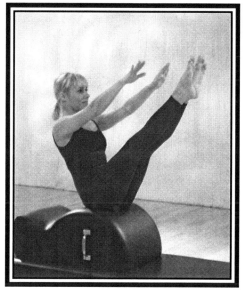 high standards would significantly decrease their applicant pool of potential apprentices.

In contrast to business tactics that dilute the integrity and effectiveness of Joseph Pilates' traditional method, it is important to understand that gaining knowledge of Pure Classical Pilates cannot be turned into a commodity for sale. It is a journey with no shortcuts, and it demands significant time, energy and work. *But the rewards are well worth one's investment.* The traditional method is an approach to integrating mental, physical and spiritual development to strengthen each facet of our existence, an approach that includes a specific pedagogy defined by Joseph Pilates, himself.

Examples of lowering training standards include:

• Reducing the number of required apprenticeship hours, sometimes to merely a weekend certification course or online certification.

• Reducing the number of direct observation hours that apprentices must complete by allowing program credit for self-study through DVDs and books.

• Changing exercises to make them easier or consumer-friendly.

• Changing exercises to fit within yoga, dance or physical therapy techniques and principles.

• Creating a simplified, factory-like formula for training apprentices.

• Hiring studio instructors from divergent training backgrounds, which can dilute teaching "culture" in a single location and reduce adherence to historical technique.

• Certifying individuals in a single apparatus, for example, the Mat, the Cadillac or the Reformer.

Compared to these examples of lowering teacher-training standards, Pure Classical Pilates is a calling in which students study and practice Joseph Pilates' traditional method—his complete system of body conditioning—for many years to become proficient practitioners and instructors.

Traditional instructors, of course, understand it is also essential to make a living as we preserve the complexity and benefits of Contrology. Yet, this road has challenging requirements of consistency, intelligence, discipline and willingness to change. These combined qualities are often not compatible with widespread consumer demand that is interested in a quick fix or a casual recreational fitness program.

There are various hidden and negative consequences to lowering training standards. One negative consequence is that naturally talented and gifted candidates will receive deficient educational training, because they stumble into the wrong teacher-certification program. It is difficult for most students to discern training programs without prior knowledge of their differences. Unfortunately, this then lowers the skill level of the entire profession. As a result of profit-driven alterations aimed at unsuspecting students and apprentices, derivative organizations often have enormous financial resources to pay for savvy, splashy advertising and worldwide training networks that mass-market substandard, diluted education.

It is unethical when an organization falsely advertises derivative training as "classical Pilates," because this claim betrays both the public's trust and its safety. Sometimes people who teach distortions of the traditional method believe they have superior knowledge compared to Joseph Pilates. Some of these individuals seem to think they are justified in re-interpreting Pure Classical Pilates. Even worse, many people believe *every* form of Pilates is valid. This dogmatic relativism corrodes Joseph Pilates' original intentions and technique. Once again, it is helpful to remember these points:

- *There is only one Pure Classical Pilates – Joseph Pilates' traditional method.*
- *There are many derivative approaches incorrectly or falsely called Pilates.*
- *"Contemporary Pilates" is a contradiction in terms.*

The traditional method is a coherent and indivisible system with infinite subtleties and innumerable modifications to accommodate various physical limitations, learning styles and aptitudes.

As an indication of how much commercial growth has occurred, there is a magazine that caters to the diverse, bustling Pilates industry. This magazine, based in New York City, makes no claim regarding preservation of Joseph Pilates' traditional method, as it covers aspects of technique, fashion, diet and travel in a reporting style all geared toward women's interests. Although the magazine lists several 1st generation instructors as part of its advisory board, its connection is tenuous with the traditional protégés of Joseph Pilates—blatantly omitting Jay Grimes—while promoting various derivative practices in an overall appeal to women's consumer interests. To this magazine's credit, however, the editors have recently published articles about Jay and Romana, which are very important for the entire profession.

Because the editors primarily sell this magazine to women, they refuse to place a photo of a man on the cover — not even a picture of Joseph Pilates himself, for fear of losing readership. The magazine also sells advertising space to individuals who market $99 teacher-certification programs. These choices do not seem to reflect the values of traditional instructors.

Pilates for Profit: The Price of Marketplace Mutation

There is no shame in entrepreneurship, big business or profit, if ethical principles and practices guide commercial activity. Most people enjoy earning a good living! The motivations of small, independent studios and self-styled industry personalities 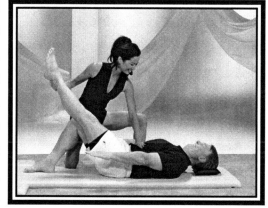 who distort Joseph Pilates' traditional method are the same as large corporations: to increase profits at the expense of preserving the method, to be creative and to differentiate their businesses in the marketplace. Large corporations, of course, can bring vast resources to bear as they expand their brand identity globally and increase their market share of sales and profits, whether it relates to the number of apprentices enrolled or amount of equipment sold.

Marketplace mutation has various forms. One relatively innocuous, yet widely adopted practice is placing studio owner names or corporate names before the word Pilates when advertising the method or technique. As hypothetical examples, consider *Jennifer's Pilates* or *John's Pilates.* It is understandable that businesses benefit from differentiating themselves from the pack, but it seems presumptuous to place the owners' names in front of Joseph Pilates' name when referring to the method itself. There is a sense of implying *possession,* as if a teacher *owned* Joseph Pilates' method or as if the business owner created *a particular style* of Pilates which, unfortunately, is true in many instances. Another person cannot possess Joseph Pilates' ideas, values and tradition. The power of the marketplace, however, has given rise to market positioning before preservation and brand building before sustaining the values and technique of Joseph Pilates' traditional method.

Not only is there a distinction to be made between how Joseph Pilates tradition is upheld in its instruction, but a salient distinction must be explained between the word "apparatus" and the word "equipment." Using the word "apparatus" should only be reserved for Joseph Pilates' designs, while the word "equipment" describes derivative machines produced by non-traditional manufacturers that distort these original designs. These untraditional machines bear little relation to Joseph Pilates' intentions or apparatus. Using his traditional studio apparatus, we are sustaining Joseph Pilates' values and practice as our bodies work *in relation to* each apparatus.

Romana would sometimes say, "Dance with your apparatus!" There is a sense that she was referring to our phenomenological experience: we are conscious of how the apparatus "partners" with us while informing and guiding our movement; we see and feel different textures of the mat, foot bar, frame and springs; and we experience the apparatus "sharing" in our timing, flow, weight, balance, length and line. The apparatus is as real and present as our consciousness of it. So, we are coordinating movement with the apparatus, as well as within ourselves.

Arguably, one of the most pernicious distortions of Joseph Pilates' traditional method stems from large derivative equipment manufacturers and their own teacher-training programs. The largest equipment manufacturers sell altered, scaled-down versions of the standard studio size traditional Universal Reformer to place in modern gyms for group Reformer classes. As a result, a single instructor may attempt to teach 10, 15, 20, 25 or more students at various levels of training and experience. Not only is it impossible to teach the foundations and nuances of Joseph Pilates' traditional technique, there is also enormous risk to the participants' safety. It is absolutely impossible for a single instructor to properly teach and correct 10, 15, 20 or 25 students simultaneously, especially with newcomers who are having their first Pilates experience. In this situation, students' ability to learn will always suffer. A new student will not receive necessary corrections, and the more advanced practitioner will be denied sufficient flow — and students of every level miss important aspects of proper placement and precision.

Chapter Six

Derivative equipment manufacturers promote their machines and teachers through the commercialization and degradation of Pure Classical Pilates in both national and international gym chains. Of course, these manufacturers do not advertise that their machines are derivative or that their businesses were founded upon distortions of Joseph Pilates' traditional system. This is a corporate lie of omission, and as a result, the public suffers from substandard teaching, hodgepodge exercise practices, and inferior equipment.

Most corporate executives have not sufficiently learned Pure Classical Pilates, and most stopped training many years ago. These individuals are, first and foremost, business professionals, physical therapists, chiropractors, and assorted other individuals who may have enjoyed the benefits of Pilates. For example, there is one businessman who originally manufactured water beds, then started making Pilates equipment when sales trends indicated a good opportunity. And instead of continuing to deepen knowledge through training, certain business owners decided to upgrade their hobby into what they hoped would be a financially lucrative career. If the directors of these training and equipment corporations actually studied the traditional method, it was often brief or piecemeal. Numerous times, I have heard someone say, "I studied with Romana," only to discover later the person had taken just one or a few lessons. Every so often there is a director who actually completed traditional training, yet who still decided to build his own derivative training organization.

I know of a large international teacher-training organization that injects substantial amounts of yoga and chiropractic principles into Joseph Pilates' traditional method. A couple of years ago, I asked the president of this derivative training organization, "With whom do you and your senior staff continue to study Pilates?" After a long pause, he replied, "We study amongst ourselves." I followed by asking, "Don't you think it would be valuable to study with a 1st-generation teacher trained by Joseph Pilates, or another principal instructor?" He replied, "Maybe one lesson." The senior training staff of this organization stopped studying Pilates in the 1980s-1990s; therefore their knowledge of the traditional method is necessarily limited. It is very sad that this company has cranked out thousands of 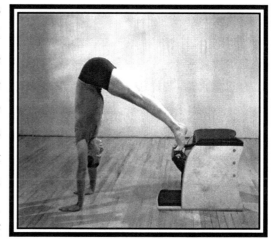 certified teachers who were trained with derivative information, incomplete knowledge and formulaic technique to accommodate a successful business formula. Here I hasten to reiterate two points: (1) students are not at fault for derivative training; and (2) there is nothing wrong with making money as long as ethical principals guide the business activity involved.

By neglect, ignorance, or duplicitous design, corporate presidents and senior training staff often steer further away from Joseph Pilates' traditional method, while sometimes falsely claiming close connections with Romana, and advertising their brand as "classical Pilates." As a result of these Pilates pyramid schemes, thousands of unwitting apprentices incorrectly presume they are learning the traditional method. When a teacher or teacher-trainer stops learning more about the traditional method, then his/her knowledge is prone to slippage or distortion. It is vital to continue studying with a traditional instructor to educate one's body in the proper ways.

As previously mentioned, program directors of derivative approaches change the traditional method to simplify and "homogenize" it to become more digestible and appealing to the masses. One supposition is that the general public is not really interested in making the commitment to properly study Joseph Pilates' traditional method; it is too difficult, it is too complex, and too expensive. I would suggest that slow, quality-controlled growth is possible and desirable in our profession.

Recall that Joseph Pilates' training sessions consisted of professional athletes and health enthusiasts who studied or practiced his method three to five days per week. His traditional work is complex, sophisticated and subtly individualized in ways that *cannot* be packaged and sold as a formula to vast numbers of people, without fundamentally simplifying the work. Loyal Romana-trained instructors remain humble and do not display contempt for Joseph Pilates' traditional method, nor do they shun the teachings of instructors who have more knowledge and experience.

It is crucial to recognize that Joseph Pilates never trained or certified instructors in a single studio apparatus. From the early days of his New York City studio through the 1990s, Mat certifications did not exist. There was no Spine Corrector certification, no Wunda Chair certification and no Reformer certification. For expediency and profit, however, self-styled industry personalities and large international corporations are doing just the opposite: they are certifying apprentices *only* in Mat exercises, then certifying apprentices *only* in Cadillac exercises and so forth.

This piecemeal approach to certification insinuates that the traditional method can be justifiably fragmented into smaller pieces. And the underlying assumption contradicts Joseph Pilates' focus upon *integrating use of all studio apparatus* in the very first lesson. Still, there exists, today, at least one large, corporate, training organization and equipment manufacturer — and many smaller organizations — that continue to dissect the method and certify apprentices in each apparatus separately.

In gym-style commercialization, I know of an international training organization and equipment manufacturer that now makes a highly distorted version of the Wunda Chair for large group classes. An instructor demonstrates exercises and plays music, so students can follow along like an aerobics class. Students who attend these classes, and who are not aware of Pure Classical Pilates, will never experience the wonderful mental and physical benefits of Joseph Pilates' traditional system. Although three of their teacher trainers studied with Romana, in my opinion, their choices constitute a betrayal of Joseph Pilates' traditional values, technique and tradition.

In contrast to the commercial gym marketing approach to business, there is yet another organization that bases its derivative technique upon physical therapy. Although the founder and director of this organization is erudite, the teachers are experienced professionals and they draw more men compared to any other organization, this group irretrievably fractures the traditional method into quasi-physical therapy and isolated movements. Individuals who comprise this organization are well-versed in physical therapy, but most do not know Joseph Pilates' traditional technique. As a result of supposed superior knowledge, these instructors exhibit little or no interest in the values and virtues of Pure Classical Pilates. Perhaps they don't know Joseph Pilates always intended for his method of Contrology to sustain and enhance "the normal healthy body" while secondarily being applicable for rehabilitation.

One very unfortunate consequence of marketing physical therapy-like Pilates simply as "Pilates" is that consumers, students and apprentices worldwide are misled into thinking Joseph Pilates' method is quasi physical therapy. In addition, I am aware of circumstances wherein teachers from this organization have promoted themselves as having superior knowledge, claiming they are more qualified Pilates instructors compared to traditionalists. Having an academic degree tends to give job applicants "an edge" when competing for jobs, but having an academic degree does not necessarily mean someone is the better candidate.

Beyond derivative styles of Pilates, we live in a modern society that promotes expediency and immediate gratification. Joseph Pilates' traditional method is not so easily achieved, so those who seek expediency or immediate gratification are bound to be disappointed. Studying the traditional method requires commitment due to the fact that progress takes consistency and hard work. Private lessons are also relatively expensive. But, if all good things are worth waiting for, certainly they are worth *working* for as well. In Pure Classical

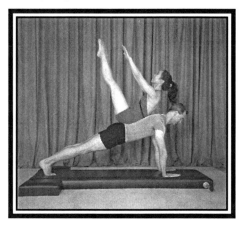

Pilates we must think and work and sweat in order to evolve. Controlled growth with the highest standards of historical accuracy and integrity is not only possible and desirable, it is already happening. Thankfully, wider recognition of the traditionalist mission is gradually, yet steadfastly, increasing.

Professions and Professional Membership

In one sense, traditional instructors are highly trained and skilled healthcare professionals. They possess considerable skill and knowledge and, therefore, warrant the recognition and pay afforded other comparable professional occupations. It could be an improvement to describe Pure Classical Pilates instructors as "professors," using the Spanish convention of naming teachers as professors, which implies their extensive training and education. The distinction of professor also denotes professional dignity and respect beyond 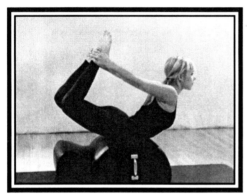 the terms "teacher" or "instructor." Becoming an accomplished traditional instructor takes about ten years of professional study, training and teaching experience. Compare ten years of professional development for accomplished traditional instructors to other professions, such as becoming an accountant, a physician, a psychologist, a computer scientist, a philosopher, business executive or pharmacist. The timeframe of professional development for all these occupations is not dissimilar.

I confess to some lament that our work isn't yet recognized as a profession that requires significant achievement, especially since our services are so essential to improving the health and well-being of countless numbers of people. In order for other professionals and the public to perceive Pure Classical Pilates instruction as a valuable occupation, on par with physical therapists, attorneys, dentists, doctors, computer scientists or university professors, it will be necessary to gradually move toward professionalization. By this, I mean the social, organizational and legal process of establishing qualifications for entry into a profession, including only those individuals who have attained the necessary knowledge or skills.

It is interesting to note that all professions, at one time in history, were trades learned by apprenticeship—just like Pilates is now—before the advent of specialized schools of education, training and state licensure. Pure Classical Pilates instructors currently work without formal professionalization, as we do not have college curricula or graduate-school training that adheres to criteria set by one of the six U.S. regional accrediting associations, although traditionalists are indeed making progress. For example, there is an excellent studio at Goucher College in Baltimore, Maryland, that sustains a high level of classical education for its students and apprentices. In looking forward, it will be valuable for colleges and universities to include an academic department—or specialization within an existing academic department—that is committed to the study and practice of Pure Classical Pilates.

Just like other professions, traditional instructors might be regulated in the future by state licensing boards, such as those for the disciplines of law, medicine, psychology and physical therapy. It will be instrumental for Pure Classical Pilates instructors to play an active role in legislative initiatives that seek to limit, or protect, our practice and livelihood. This way, we have a better chance at preserving Joseph Pilates' values and technique.

Chapter Six

At present, we do not have a single professional membership organization that represents our values, skills, educational standards and mission to preserve Joseph Pilates' traditional method. Membership organizations can be useful to create a public identity, to share knowledge, and to influence the outcome of beneficial legislative initiatives. In discussions with colleagues, however, some people question the value of establishing an organization of traditionalists, because there are inevitable policy conflicts, vested interests, political maneuvering and, of course, membership dues. Then our work might become more about formulating policies, procedures, meetings and business matters than devoting our time to teaching or studying. Even though traditionalists do not have a formal organization, we have the worldwide Academy Directory on www.ClassicalPilates.net for networking, training, collaborating and locating referrals from a trusted source.

Although traditionalists do not currently have an organization that represents our interests, there is one large membership group that questionably claims to act on behalf of all instructors. In my view, this group is too eclectic to represent traditional instructors. This membership group has proclaimed itself to be "The United Nations of Pilates," while supposedly preserving Joseph Pilates' tradition, which is a poignant contradiction in terms. It is not possible to preserve Joseph Pilates' traditional method, while simultaneously accepting and promoting various deviations of Joseph Pilates' indivisible system.

This membership organization supports divergent styles of Pilates, promotes its annual conferences, and administers a multiple-choice examination wherein practitioners can become "certified" without assessment of their teaching skills and without passing verbal or written examinations. This group is contradictorily attempting to position itself as a type of *commercial* licensing board— which exhibits an inherent conflict of interest—that tries to establish educational standards for the industry while simultaneously "certifying" instructors. No other professional membership organization (for example, American Medical Association or American Psychological Association) serves the 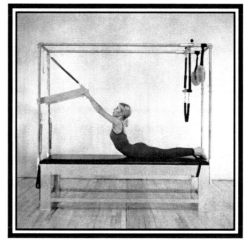 dual role of promoting the best interests of its members while granting a license to practice, or in this case a certification. Only state licensing boards have the authority to examine applicants for their legal privilege to provide professional services.

Beyond membership organizations, numerous commercial conventions and trade shows promote a variety of derivative styles of Pilates and other forms of body conditioning. Some traditionalists attend and teach at these large-scale conferences, because it can be beneficial to share our knowledge of Joseph Pilates' traditional system with other teachers and the public.

Throughout the world, traditionalists are much smaller in number compared to derivative instructors, so it is not easy to find common values at the large trade-show conventions. Having said this, however, it can be beneficial for traditionalists to periodically attend and teach at these commercial events, to see the larger commercial world of Pilates, to learn about business, and to help promote Joseph Pilates' traditional technique in the world. Hold fast to your values and enter the world.

Gender Imbalance yet Equal Opportunity

Today, almost all Pilates students and instructors are women. In Joseph Pilates' original studio, the gender ratio was exactly opposite. In today's world of physical fitness, men generally stay in shape by "typically male" modes of exercise: lifting weights, running, basic calisthenics or team sports, as well as a variety of other activities including skiing, swimming, track and field events, snow boarding, surfing, skate boarding and so forth.

When Joseph Pilates came to the United States in the 1920s, his studio was occupied by men. He trained pugilists, circus performers and health enthusiasts. He purposely located his studio close to the old Madison Square Garden in New York City to train boxers. So, why has there been a complete reversal in the gender ratio of those who train in Pure Classical Pilates? One reason is that during the 1930s, 1940s and 1950s, increasing numbers of professional dancers, most of them women, began studying with Joseph and Clara Pilates. As the gender ratio changed to reflect increased participation by women, perhaps men began perceiving Joseph's traditional method as an activity primarily *for* women. As a result of this gender shift in Joseph Pilates' studio, as well as the influence of cultural expectations for both genders, men gradually began to seek out more stereotypically male-oriented workout settings such as gymnasiums and sports clubs.

Given the many comments Kathy, Romana and Jay have made about Joseph Pilates, this gender shift disappointed him. Joseph Pilates' work was originally influenced by the energy and exercises of gymnastics and calisthenics; yet, his method became subtly, but increasingly misinterpreted by the dancers who sought out his instruction. Kathy, Romana and Jay have all said Joseph Pilates did not like teaching dancers for this reason. As time passed, certain movement qualities associated with dancers and conventional femininity began to supersede movement qualities associated with non-dancers and conventional masculinity.

> **Joseph Pilates rightfully believed proper physical conditioning occasions optimal mental functioning.**

In general, as more women dancers began to teach the method, there was increased emphasis on counting repetitions and refined aspects of movement, such as poise, long beautiful lines and graceful strength. Although some of these movement qualities were certainly part of Joseph Pilates' traditional method, other more "masculine" aspects of gymnastic strength, vigor and abrupt stop-start exercises are practiced less often nowadays.

This gender shift compounded Joseph Pilates' long-term discouragement that his method of body conditioning was never fully recognized — during his lifetime — as a valuable and legitimate system of preventative medicine and rehabilitation in the medical community, or in the public at large. As Joseph Pilates said himself, "I am 50 years ahead of my time." Kathy Grant commented about times when Joseph Pilates

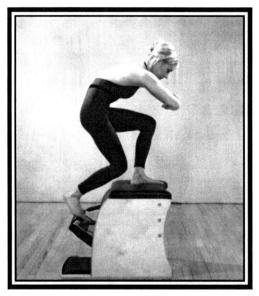

seemed despondent, and Clara would gently comfort him.

In contrast to his disappointment, Joseph Pilates gained a solid reputation among small groups of the world's most successful athletes and dancers, as well as many celebrity singers and actors. The famous ballet choreographer George Balanchine studied with Joseph Pilates and referred dancers to him regularly. In fact, Balanchine paid Joseph Pilates royalties for certain Contrology movements used in the production of "The Seven Deadly Sins," featuring Allegra Kent.

In more recent times, even greater distortions of the traditional method have emerged along gender lines. There are studios in which owners radically change the traditional method by "feminizing" the studio into a spa atmosphere with soft music, candles, pink wall paint, or assorted meditation-like movements that bear no resemblance to Joseph Pilates' New York City studio and strong conditioning system.

Although nothing is inherently wrong with these aesthetic choices, they are at odds with the spirit of Joseph Pilates' teachings, and they distract from his intentions that body conditioning should be a strong muscular workout. The addition of various softer accessories and delicate movement influences has only furthered an already growing disparity between men and women practitioners. In contrast to the feminization of some studio environments, there are indeed hundreds of accomplished women instructors listed in the www.ClassicalPilates.net Academy Directory who teach Joseph Pilates' strong method the way he intended, without softening the studio environment or changing his exercises.

Another reason for the dearth of men studying Pilates is that gender identification in the fitness world goes far beyond instruction in the studio to how it is marketed and advertised. Pilates advertising on television, in magazines, and in health clubs is almost entirely geared toward women's interests. Women probably own 99% of studios in the world, as well as manage 99% of the teacher-training programs. Pilates is a female dominated occupation.

Could there be another source for this stark gender ratio difference? Enter psychology, gender identity and self-worth: the Pilates profession does not have significant occupational stature, nor does it offer financial incentives relatively equal to the fields of law, business, medicine, finance, real estate, banking, computer technology, pharmaceuticals and so forth. In most societies, men are still primarily valued for their financial earning power, occupational status or access to financial wealth. So, it is understandable that most men are not interested in becoming traditional instructors. These conventional markers of success—and our profession's lack of them—affect recruitment efforts to attract more men to the Pure Classical Pilates fold. In spite of these cultural, psychological and financial obstacles, there is a small minority of disciplined and talented men who are devoted to Pure Classical Pilates. Perhaps one day the Pilates profession will gain enough occupational significance in society to offer increased employee salaries and benefits to both women and men.

To expand the Pilates "brotherhood," I make these suggestions to help encourage more men to study and train in the traditional Pilates method:

- Communicate Joseph Pilates' biographical history to students, apprentices and the public. He was a gymnast, boxer and all-around athlete, whose athleticism was enhanced by his commitment to developing mind, body and spirit through Contrology.

- Host Pilates workshops specifically for men, focusing on aspects of strength, coordination and skill and then relate these qualities to running, golf, swimming, football, basketball, tennis, surfing, skiing, snow boarding and so forth.

- Actively recruit men to become instructors.

- Include photos of men in studio advertisements and testimonials of men in brochures, books and DVDs.

- Buy, read and sell Daniel Lyon's book *The Complete Book of* Pilates *for Men* (HarperCollins 2005).

- Develop professional connections within college and university academic departments, medical practices, and establish a traditional Pilates association that represents our best interests to keep educational standards high and legislative initiatives favorable.

My hope is that traditional instructors and other allied healthcare professionals will encourage more men to pursue careers as Pure Classical Pilates instructors. We welcome newcomers with open arms so we and can all enjoy the wonderful experience of Pure Classical Pilates together. To share the words of Kathy Grant, the esteemed master teacher, "The Pilates method was made for men."

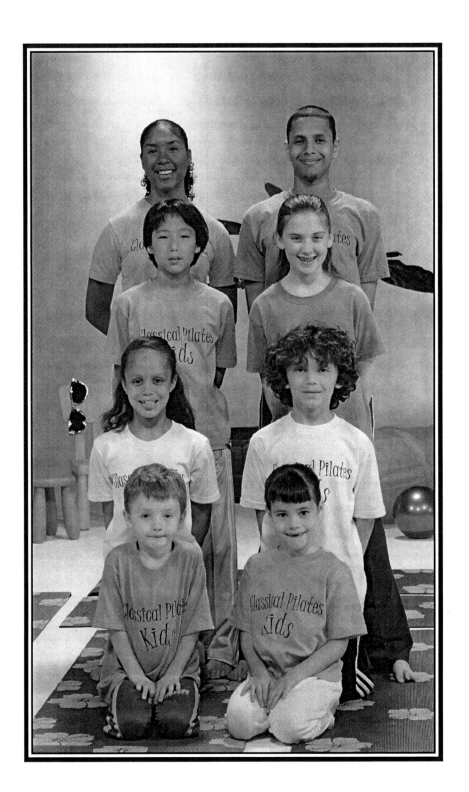

Chapter 7

Keeping the Tradition Alive

Chapter Seven

Traditional instructors may seem outnumbered by the purveyors of derivative approaches, but, collectively, we are a vibrant and active force teaching Pure Classical Pilates around the world. By teaching students, managing studios and educating the public, hundreds, if not thousands, of loyal instructors have been keeping Joseph Pilates' traditional method alive. It is vital that dedicated traditionalists seek opportunities to preserve and grow their discipline. It is imperative that traditional instructors create interesting ways to collaborate with one another, teach continuing education workshops, write more books, make more instructional DVDs, and offer more presentations to the public and to other professionals. Perhaps most importantly, those of us devoted to Joseph Pilates' traditional method should make some commitment, large or small, to share this knowledge with a new generation of teachers.

I love the traditional method and continue to work toward the growth and expansion of this valuable tradition — and perhaps you, the reader, will also take up this cause. This chapter describes a few ways that I have been personally involved in helping preserve the traditional method. In doing so, I hope to inspire others to continue teaching and enjoying new interesting ways to educate the public about Pure Classical Pilates.

There are many aspects of my work, including but not limited to: teaching students and instructors and providing continuing education credits; sustaining the free Academy Directory of traditional instructors and teacher training programs listed on www.ClassicalPilates.net, which helps promote our collective interests; producing the *Classical Pilates Technique* series of six instructional DVDs; and helping coordinate individual workshops and conferences, nationally and internationally, that preserve and promote Joseph Pilates' traditional method.

The Worldwide Academy of Traditionalists

Lineage is essential. To help preserve Joseph Pilates' traditional method and prevent its deterioration by derivative approaches, I maintain the worldwide Academy Directory of traditional instructors, who have demonstrated their dedication to teaching the traditional method with integrity and accuracy. Our lineage sources directly from Joseph and Clara Pilates. Currently, there are more than 1,000 professionals—in effect, a worldwide faculty of Pure Classical Pilates professors—listed in the Directory. The Academy Directory includes: (1) independent studios *without* training programs; (2) independent studios *with* training programs; and (3) multi-studio training organizations.

There is no fee for being listed in the Academy Directory. Although every best effort is made to keep contact information updated, I do ask for your help! Should you find inaccurate information listed, please send your updates. Keep in mind, this remains a community service to help preserve and promote Joseph Pilates' traditional method and heritage.

Chapter Seven

If you are new to Pilates, please practice due diligence and confirm first that your instructor continues to teach the traditional method. It is generally safe to assume most Academy Directory members are "keepers of the flame." Students may notice, however, that each instructor has different teaching nuances. Overall, however, we share a common purpose of preserving Joseph Pilates' values and technique, imparting instruction, examining apprentices, and promoting education in the science and athletic art of his traditional method.

I recommend that students and teachers of every school avail themselves of Academy Directory instructors to gain more knowledge and experience in Pure Classical Pilates. As I mentioned before, *you are welcome to study with traditionalists and, one day, become one of us.* The worldwide Academy Directory of traditionalists is not a single institution. It is a network of teaching and training facilities with shared values that, taken collectively, guide students and prepare graduates for responsible teaching and leadership in the profession. At locations all around the globe, Academy Directory members provide various group classes, private and semi-private instruction to students, as well as individualized training courses and a variety of flexible enrollment options for apprentices.

Policies and requirements vary depending upon the studio and training program; yet, the minimum number of required apprentice hours is 600–1,000+, in addition to regularly training with a supervising instructor. Collectively, we provide experience-based education to students. There are no Internet certifications or online certifications. And there are no certifications solely based upon a multiple-choice written examination, as in the case of the membership organization I previously mentioned.

In contrast to derivative training programs that include movement mixed with other disciplines, Academy Directory members offer pure, comprehensive training and support to those who want to become traditional instructors. Many apprentices have already had another career in sports, gymnastics, business, law, track and field or dance. Many apprentices have completed college, professional school or graduate school before admission to a rigorous traditional teacher training program. Suffice it to say that Academy Directory members are accomplished individuals.

Teacher training programs in the worldwide Academy Directory emphasize the development of technical facility, communication skills, critical thinking, and individualized teaching according to the aptitudes, limitations and perceived limitations of each student. Teacher trainers also encourage apprentices to explore — and strike a balance between — training, teaching and the fundamental principles of Joseph Pilates' traditional method.

Traditional instructors understand the importance of honesty and respect in preserving the integrity of Joseph Pilates' traditional method, as well as how practicing and safeguarding the work occasions people to become better citizens in society. Sustaining proficiency through practice and study in Pure Classical Pilates fortifies commitment in our worldwide educational community. In turn, these values improve health and well-being, and contribute positively to our functioning in the world. If we are relatively physically fit and mentally well-adjusted, then we aspire to live with purpose regarding work, love, family, friends and society.

Academy Directory instructors are grounded in the roots of Joseph Pilates' true method; we stand firm with the trunk of the tree of knowledge; we branch out toward the future with our own distinct voices; we are the stewards who have been entrusted to carry on the virtues and values of Pure Classical Pilates, which have collectively comprised the highest standards of excellence for fulfilling Joseph Pilates' original educational mission.

> **The intention and integrity of Joseph Pilates' traditional system occasions people to become better citizens in society.**

Let It Be: Rewriting Tradition Rewards No One

Over 1,000 Romana-trained instructors and teacher trainers—as well as their own 3rd generation graduates—continue to preserve Pure Classical Pilates with skill, passion, loyalty and athletic artfulness. There are also several instructors listed in the Academy Directory who trained with Kathy Grant.

As a friendly reminder, Romana and Jay would often say Joseph Pilates' traditional method was "made for the normal, healthy body." Although we can debate what a normal healthy body is until the "end of infinity," Joseph Pilates' archival films clearly show him working with uninjured, relatively healthy students. Both Romana and Jay have loyally carried Joseph Pilates' work forward, and now it is our responsibility to protect this legacy.

Romana often says that when teachers get bored with their work, they will surely change the traditional Pilates method. Thus, to prevent boredom or burnout, I suggest continuing your own study of the traditional method with teachers who keep you inspired, and cultivate other physical activities independent of Pilates. For example, try swimming, basketball, football, 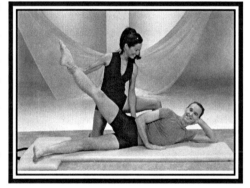 walking, skateboarding, skiing, tennis, ballroom dancing, sky diving, scuba diving—anything that invigorates you! Another possibility is to find or create a completely different part-time career to remain energized and balanced while teaching traditional Pilates. Remember, the traditional method inspires balance, so we should strive for balance in our lives. Make every effort not to burn out! The world needs traditional instructors and Joseph Pilates' traditional system of conditioning.

Chapter Seven

Some instructors change the historically accurate method when they haven't fully understood it, or when they haven't mastered the work. Of course, no one ever completely masters Joseph Pilates' traditional method. There is *always* room for learning and improvement. It is relatively easy to devise new exercises, as well as create new exercise orders. Yet attempting to "reinvent the wheel" to prevent boredom or burnout will invariably expend wasted energy toward futile and pointless goals. Joseph Pilates' traditional method is sufficiently complex and sophisticated to sustain a lifetime of interest and exhilaration, while we work toward new disclosures of meaning, new understandings of movement, as well as new realms of body-mind evolution. There are indeed enough modifications within the traditional method to comprise infinite variety, especially when you consider each student possesses a unique combination of mental and physical aptitudes.

These days, I hear people who say new knowledge requires us to change Pure Classical Pilates. These days, I hear that it's okay to simplify or abbreviate Joseph Pilates' traditional method in order to market it to the masses. These days, I hear people say Joseph Pilates would have evolved and changed his own method. Perhaps, but if Joseph Pilates felt his technique could be improved, or his method could be adapted to the changing whims of culture, it is likely he would have included in his original instruction a provision to do either, or both.

Pure Classical Pilates on Film:
A Quest to Capture the Magic

In 1996, I decided to become an apprentice at The Pilates Studio in New York City, and I began studying weekly with master instructor Romana Kryzanowska at Drago's Gym from 1997–2002. Every Friday at 11:00 am was my time to journey with Romana into the realm of hard work, sweat, good fun and athletic artistry. Studying with Romana was a precious gift. I was in the presence of greatness. Romana possesses much more than knowledge of the traditional method. She is the essence of elegance; she sees with piercing perceptiveness; she speaks with insightful humor and shares her abundant love of life with students. Romana can also sparkle with a galaxy of magic and a trace of mischief, as she finds subtle ways of helping students discover wonderful qualities in themselves. Romana also brings forth Joseph Pilates' spirit, his discipline and his understanding of what is — or should be — important in our lives. When Romana is teaching, you are deeply connected to Joseph Pilates' spirit and traditional work.

After each lesson I expressed my gratitude to Romana, knowing my spoken appreciation paled in comparison to her wonderful gifts of teaching. Romana periodically replied, "Why are you thanking me? I'm just passing on what Uncle Joe taught me." Romana's sincerity and deep humility showed her true colors. This absolutely wonderful and brilliant protégé of Joseph Pilates was simply describing herself as a loyal messenger.

Chapter Seven

In 2000, Romana asked three instructors to demonstrate Mat workouts in her first commercial DVD project. Being invited was indeed a humbling experience, as well as an honor, because we were helping preserve Joseph Pilates' traditional method with Romana. Yet, she did not have control over the directing or editing, which is absolutely necessary to capture good technique on film. Understanding and teaching Pure Classical Pilates is one endeavor; it is a totally different job to film the traditional work while demonstrating its integrity, precision and spirit.

After completing this project, Romana made it clear on several occasions she did not like filming the traditional method. Although she never explained why, my sense is that Romana believed filming the method simplifies its complexity and athletic artfulness. In a real sense, the traditional Pilates method is necessarily compromised on film and we are left with an inferior depiction. It is an elusive endeavor to capture all the dimensions, energy and intense muscular action of Pure Classical Pilates on film, because movement qualities are subtle and cannot always be discriminated by the viewer's eye. These same movement qualities, however, can be clearly perceptible when experienced by the student and seen by the trained eyes of an instructor.

Even so, I began to feel a growing sense of urgency to document Joseph Pilates' remarkable creation on film, because the industry was growing so rapidly. Derivative approaches were hastily expanding and spreading like viruses. So, one day, I asked Romana if she would direct a

DVD to preserve the traditional method with students of her choosing. Romana graciously gave me her consent to pursue my own project and granted use of her name for a dedication, but she declined to participate, citing her agreement with The Pilates Studio in New York City. I thanked Romana for her generosity and began to think about how to begin this project. The series of six *Classical Pilates Technique* DVDs, described at the back of this book, was the result.

In the beginning, I never intended to sell a single DVD. My purpose was to document Joseph Pilates' traditional method on film, which was so it would not get lost to the increasing jungle of derivative influences quickly gaining popularity.

Originally, I thought a few other instructors might be interested in having a copy. After I produced the first video, which was just a simple visual "outline" of the traditional method, many instructors asked for copies. I gladly gave away many videos as mementos. Soon, as 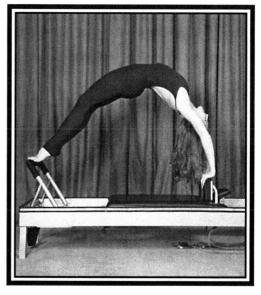 more and more requests flooded in, it was clear there was a much greater need I had not initially realized.

Due to family and organizational dynamics, Romana sensed it would be difficult to continue teaching me.

She lovingly said, "It's time for you to spread your wings. All birds must fly away. You know the method; the method is in you; it's time for you to fly." Romana conveyed her words with love and kindness. Yet, I understood their darker implication, which was heartbreaking. Over the years, her decision has occasioned currents of sorrow, but I am not the only one. There are many loyal instructors who dearly love and revere Romana, and who keep the method pure. These instructors have also found themselves in similar circumstances. Not too long ago, I spoke with Romana over the phone and met with her personally. She was as lovely and gracious as ever. She asked if I would like to schedule a lesson sometime. Of course! In retrospect, perhaps one immanent goal of a teacher — or parent — is to guide a student to a place where her role as a teacher is no longer needed.

Proclaiming the Importance of Joseph Pilates' Original Tradition

It is rare that someone will contact me asking where he can train with a qualified instructor of the traditional method. The fact remains that most people will seek exercise that is economical, and convenient, with less consideration given to the quality and professional standards. I readily understand this impulse, as I too am a consumer of many things: transportation, food, clothing, communication, office products and so forth. Convenience is important. There are areas I am willing to compromise, but when it comes to my education and health, I seek only that which will meet my needs best, regardless of ease or cost. Likewise, if a student does value the traditional method, traditional instructors are indeed worthy of such investment.

Traditional instructors do not have an equal voice in the larger commercialized arena of derivative approaches. The primary reason is that Pure Classical Pilates teachers place importance upon studying, training, teaching and preserving the work. Yes, of course, we manage studios and promote our businesses, but these activities do not exceed our commitment to preserving and teaching the traditional work. We are devoted to Joseph Pilates' traditional method, to Romana's teachings and to Jay's teachings. Even though traditional instructors might be less intensely focused on marketing their businesses, we are growing in number and beginning to share our collective knowledge with the world. In spite of some differences within the "family" of traditional instructors, we have much larger obstacles to overcome as we engage Joseph Pilates' heritage in the wider profession.

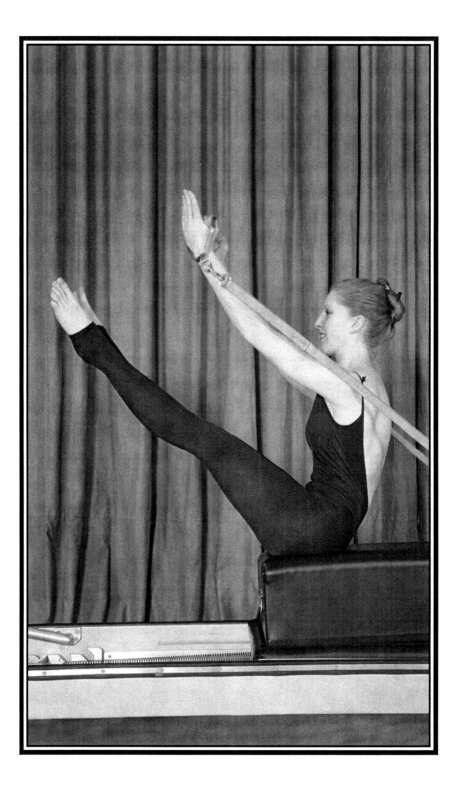

Chapter 8

Standards of Excellence:
Studio Conduct, Basic Tips
and a Proposed Code of Ethics

Chapter Eight

Studios that teach the traditional method are unique. Ideally, they honor Joseph Pilates' tradition while inculcating deference and propriety. These traditional studios possess high standards of excellence. Collectively, they respect the oral communication of Joseph Pilates' teachings and are wholeheartedly committed to his indivisible classical technique.

In traditional studios, the ego is checked at the front door! Students are expected to put forth full effort with teachers who are challenging and demanding, yet still pleasant and encouraging. Although there is a virtual playground of creative interesting work within the athletic art of Joseph Pilates' traditional method, student-teacher relations are not democratic. Students should respect the tradition and adapt to the traditional method in order to gain the best benefits of health and well-being.

Conduct in the Traditional Studio

People who have been involved in gymnastics, martial arts, organized sports or dance are familiar with the protocols of their disciplines. If you have a previous movement background, these experiences transfer to the protocols of a traditional studio. If someone has not had previous training in another physically oriented discipline, it is possible to be unprepared. For example, new students arrive at their lesson and sometimes place their backpacks, gym bags, grocery bags, book bags, purses or briefcases directly on traditional apparatus. This is unhygienic and inappropriate, because the bottom of any carry bag is dirty. It is important that traditional studios sustain a proper level of cleanliness, especially because we place our arms, legs and faces on the apparatus during a workout.

When people place carry bags, shopping bags or purses on traditional apparatus, they lack consideration for the safety and hygiene of others. Second, they are unaware of different conventions that may apply to the traditional studio. In any new situation, it is prudent to act in a respectful manner by asking questions about proper decorum. The same idea applies to people who sit, recline or stand on the apparatus while wearing street clothes, which might also be unclean from work and normal daily use. Believe it or not, I have seen many uninitiated people do exactly this after entering a traditional studio. So, please do not wear street clothes while sitting or lying down on traditional apparatus.

There is another important rule in traditional studios: for safety reasons, students should not begin using an apparatus without direct supervision by an instructor, unless they have prior approval for a solo workout after at least 30+ private lessons. Pure Classical Pilates is challenging, and it is possible to get injured. To cite my own experience, I have accidentally fallen completely off the Reformer — to the floor — after my hand slipped while practicing the Front Split exercise. In another case, I accidentally fell down on the Reformer carriage demonstrating the Snake/Twist, because my hand slipped off the shoulder block. In yet another surprise, my foot slipped off the foot bar doing Semi-Circle. Over the years, I have seen other experienced instructors slip and fall off different apparatus. Students should, therefore, be accompanied and taught by an instructor.

Students also need guidance to properly learn the traditional method. It is important to correct bad habits

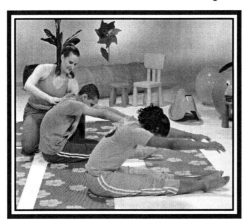 and increase technical proficiency. On numerous occasions, I have seen students with insufficient training start using traditional apparatus before their instructor arrives. This is unsafe and students will not receive the benefit of instruction to correctly learn the traditional method.

Another area of studio propriety is the standard 24-hour cancellation policy. If you cancel your appointment within 24 hours of the designated time, then you should pay for the entire lesson, no matter the reason. Though it is a standard set by almost every other profession, many students, unfortunately, do not always respect this policy. Oftentimes, students ask their teacher — or office manager — to forfeit the late-cancellation fee. Students should consider that instructors make their living by teaching Pure Classical Pilates, and studio owners must pay their instructors for a late-cancelled hour. In order to encourage students to carefully consider their priorities and respect an instructor's time the same way one would a physician, dentist or an attorney, students will be charged for a late-cancelled appointment.

The Ideal World Checklist:
Pure Classical Pilates Do's and Don'ts

Traditional Instructors DO:

- Obtain proper education and certification (at least 600–1,000+ apprenticeship hours) through training programs listed in the Pure Classical Pilates Academy Directory.
- Seek continuing education through lessons and workshops.
- Refer to the proposed code of ethics in *Discovering Pure Classical Pilates* that aims to protect students' best interests and well-being.
- Respect the original values, principles and technique developed by Joseph Pilates.
- Refer students to an appropriate medical specialist if a student's condition or symptoms warrant a second opinion or treatment.
- Use only traditional Pilates apparatus.
- Promote the values, principles and technique of Joseph Pilates' traditional method through one or more avenues, such as teaching, writing, speaking, publishing, advertising and organizing workshops.
- Use common sense with regard to safety and teaching.

Traditional Instructors DO NOT:

- Offer single-apparatus certification, including Mat certification, or recommend derivative distortions.
- Significantly alter traditional technique and standard modifications to satisfy misplaced outlets for creativity, boredom or unwarranted student requests.
- Practice or create derivative, hybrid, commercialized Pilates techniques.

Traditional Students DO:

- Seek education and certification (at least 600–1,000+ apprenticeship hours) through training programs listed in the Academy Directory.
- Study with instructors who have traditional training, education and apparatus.
- Develop an active learning approach by asking questions.
- Use common sense with regard to safety and training.
- Have an initial understanding of the proposed traditional instructor's code of ethics.

Traditional Students DO NOT:

- Enroll in single-apparatus certification courses or become affiliated with derivative organizations.

- Practice derivative approaches of the traditional method.
- Wear inappropriate attire, use derivative apparatus or resource material for training and education.
- Study with instructors without first researching their background and training to establish their professional adequacy.
- Sacrifice historically accurate technique for derivative exercises that feel "easier" or "better."

Pure Classical Pilates: A Proposed Code of Ethics

Throughout history, groups of individuals who share common values, actions or purposes have created codes of conduct or codes of ethics. From military personnel to religious orders; from medical professionals to journalists; and from international treaties between nations to private fraternal organizations, developing a sound code of ethics helps guide everyday professional activities and addresses uncertainties when ethical dilemmas arise.

The ethical guidelines below were adapted from three organizations (American Society of Exercise Physiologists, American Psychological Association, and IDEA Health & Fitness Association). They comprise a tentative proposal, a beginning point for instructors, to discuss the merits and limitations of these conditions and refine the concepts over time.

ACCORD

1. Instructors are of good moral character and strive to benefit their students. Instructors also take care to do no harm.
2. Instructors establish relationships of trust with students, colleagues and other professionals.

COMPETENCE & FAIR ACCESS

3. Instructors are highly trained practitioners and educators of Joseph Pilates' traditional method, and they are responsible for professional competence in practice and teaching.
4. Instructors provide instruction in the practice of body conditioning, in addition to communicating knowledge related to educational, preventive, rehabilitative, and/or research services equitably to all individuals, regardless of social or economic status, age, gender, race, ethnicity, national origin, religion, disability, diverse values, attitudes or opinions.

EDUCATION

5. Instructors have at least 600 hours of apprenticeship with a traditional 1st or 2nd generation instructor, and they should maintain high quality professional competence through continued education.
6. Instructors are encouraged to give traditional Pilates method workshops and lessons to various

professionals in the field, including specialists in health and fitness, preventive medicine, rehabilitation, education and research.

7. Instructors respect and protect the privacy, rights, and confidentiality of all individuals by not disclosing student information, unless required by law or when confidentiality jeopardizes the health and safety of others.

INSTRUCTION

8. Instructors provide appropriate modifications of exercises that allow for individual variation in aptitude, limitation and previous experience.

9. Instructors recommend products or services only if they will benefit a student's health and well-being, not because they will benefit them or their employer financially or occupationally.

10. Instructors choose exercises for individuals and groups based upon traditional technique, safety, effectiveness. They do not allow creativity to compromise traditional technique, safety or effectiveness.

SCOPE OF SERVICES

11. Instructors provide services and teach only within the boundaries of their competence, based on their education, training, supervised experience, consultation, study, or professional

experience; therefore, instructors only work within the scope of their knowledge and skill. When necessary, they refer students to another professional for consultation.

ACCOUNTABILITY

12. Instructors are concerned about the ethical compliance of their colleagues' professional conduct. Instructors informally resolve such issues by bringing them to the attention of the individual in question or a supervisor.

13. Instructors contribute to the ongoing development and integrity of the profession by being responsive, mutually supportive, and accurately communicating academic and other qualifications to colleagues and associates in health and fitness, preventive, rehabilitative, educational and/or research services and programs.

PROFESSIONALISM

14. Instructors do not exploit persons over whom they have supervisory, evaluative or other authority such as students, supervisees and employees.

15. When instructors provide teaching services, they obtain the informed consent of the individual or individuals using language that is reasonably understandable to that person or persons, except when conducting such activities without consent is mandated by law or governmental regulation.

16. Instructors do not engage in sexual harassment. Sexual harassment is sexual solicitation, physical advances, or verbal or nonverbal conduct that is sexual in nature, that occurs in connection with the instructor's activities or role as an instructor, and that either (a) is unwelcome, is offensive, or creates a hostile workplace or educational environment, and the instructor knows or is told this; or (b) is sufficiently severe or intense to be abusive to a reasonable person in the context. Sexual harassment can consist of a single intense or severe act or of multiple persistent or pervasive acts.

17. Termination of Services: (a) Instructors may terminate teaching or training services when it becomes reasonably clear that the student (or apprentice) no longer needs the service, is not likely to benefit, or is being harmed by continued service; (b) Instructors may terminate instruction when threatened or otherwise endangered by the student or another person with whom the student has a relationship; (c) Except where precluded by the actions of students or third-party payers, prior to termination, instructors provide sufficient pre-termination notice and suggest alternative service providers as appropriate.

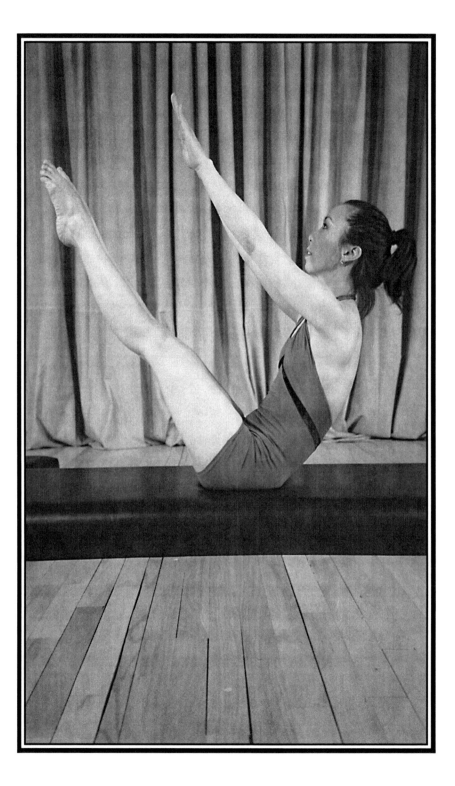

Epilogue

Epilogue

A Call for a Return to the Classics

To truly understand and proficiently teach Joseph Pilates' traditional method, it takes many years of study, practice and continued training. As I have previously described, it is important to conceptualize Joseph Pilates' traditional method as *a unique and indivisible system;* meaning, there is coherence and order to the exercises, each resonating with others, none working against others. The progression of each exercise forms an epigenetic sequence. That is, each set of exercises builds on and requires mastery of the preceding set.

To honor the work of Joseph Pilates' essential contribution to health and well-being, we should continue to learn, grow and evolve within the traditional method. This way we can optimally achieve the increased vitality, balance, strength and coordination that he intended. Those who consider Pure Classical Pilates as a type of recreational exercise, self-help activity, or simply the most recent fitness fad cannot fully realize its value. It is precisely because Joseph Pilates' work aims toward coordinating body, mind, and spirit — through extensive movement vocabulary and ordered sequences — that we can distinguish the traditional method from generic body conditioning, general exercise training, and consumer-oriented recreational fitness trends.

Fitness instructors, or various other body conditioning professionals, may be skeptical of how or why Joseph Pilates' traditional method warrants such extensive training. To those of you who may think teaching Pure Classical Pilates is not a true profession, and the training necessary is not worth the time, effort, and money, and you believe that traditional instructors do not make a significant effect in the lives of others . . . you're wrong! How do I know for sure? Because I've done both. And I'm here to tell you that not only is teaching as worthwhile as my profession as a psychologist, and my training just as grueling, but it is especially so in my ability to make a positive effect in the lives of others.

To many people, the prospect of going through extensive training to become a traditional instructor may seem, at best, overly involved and, at worst, a bad investment. After all, why work so diligently to become proficient in teaching Pure Classical Pilates, when the monetary rewards are relatively modest? The answer is that we are healthcare professionals who have a commitment to helping others realize their full potential as human beings.

There are hundreds, if not thousands, of naturally gifted instructors. As healthcare professionals, we guide others toward health and well-being, while we preserve the knowledge and skill of Joseph Pilates' traditional system. It is the love of Pure Classical Pilates, the extensive education, the passion to develop professional skill, and the exuberance of sharing this work with others that define members in the Academy Directory as "keepers of the flame."

Academy Directory members are indeed a worldwide "family" that share the same values regarding Pure Classical Pilates. We look deeply into the traditional method for a good workout and, even more deeply, for self-analysis, growth,

Epilogue

healing and a return to wholeness. Joseph Pilates' traditional method also helps us cope with problems in everyday living. Traditionalists naturally continue studying and training with Academy Directory teacher trainers. As a worldwide family, it is detrimental to be divided by secondary conflicts between us. We are charged with the much larger and more important mission of remaining positive, supporting one another, and sharing our knowledge with the world.

As traditionalists share their knowledge with others, interesting situations arise. It has been my experience that when non-traditionalist instructors begin to study Pure Classical Pilates, they frequently become invigorated—even hungry—to learn more about the traditional method as they begin to experience its extraordinary benefits. These instructors sometimes have frustration and disappointment because their previous derivative Pilates training cannot be adequately compared to Joseph Pilates' traditional method.

In contrast to derivative approaches, the value and benefits of Joseph Pilates' indivisible system cannot be overstated: we simply achieve better mind-body coordination, increased alertness, preparedness for action or emergencies, improved posture, prevention of injuries and improved self-esteem, to name just a few benefits. Derivative approaches are not capable of providing all the remarkable health benefits of Joseph Pilates' traditional method, nor can their teacher-training programs screen apprentices for devotion and passion. These two elements are found with loyal instructors listed in the Academy Directory.

There is good news amidst the clanging cacophony of derivative approaches: many potential students and apprentices are starting to "separate the wheat from the chaff," by asking specific questions to identify the most qualified instructors. Prospective students and apprentices are seeking answers to questions like these:

- *Which teacher-training program did my teacher attend?*
- *Did my instructor complete comprehensive training?*
- *Which approach or style of Pilates did my teacher study?*
- *How many hours of apprenticeship were involved?*
- *How many years of teaching experience does my instructor have?*
- *Is the studio affiliated with a particular training program?*
- *Is so, which one?*

These can be useful questions to ask the studio owner or supervising instructor where you are studying.

Fanning the Flame:
The Future of Pure Classical Pilates

Now that you have discovered essential dimensions of Pure Classical Pilates, go forward and use these insights to educate and integrate your body, mind and spirit with vigorous enthusiasm!

For everyone — newcomers, students, enthusiasts, teachers and teacher trainers — I strongly recommend continuing on the path of Pure Classical Plates technique, because you gain the most comprehensive mental and physical benefits from Joseph Pilates' traditional method. Take advantage of the Academy Directory and pursue the best available training.

If seekers of the light and keepers of the flame come together—open of heart, pure of intention and respectful of custom—the Pure Classical Pilates experience can be a warm one, burning calories while blazing trails toward a healthier mind and spirit!

As we look forward, we should understand the future of Pure Classical Pilates rests in the hands of loyal traditionalists who teach the traditional method with love and skillfulness. We are the inheritors of Joseph Pilates' hallowed tradition because we work for it, we preserve it, and we share it with the world. After all, this is what Romana, Jay and Kathy have done over the decades. Let us continue to enjoy "living the movement," as we share the responsibility for carrying Pure Classical Pilates forward to future generations with strength and grace. As Romana would say, "If you are true to Pilates, Pilates will be true to you."

Joseph Pilates, the master himself, passed his torch to very few dedicated and faithful protégés. Their work over the decades has fanned the flames of our knowledge, tradition and individual transformation. I have faith the pure work will continue to grow as it is increasingly understood and practiced by the public.

I hope you, too, keep the flames strong as you live that light of inspiration for future generations.

Epilogue

References

Adler, Mortimer J. (1982) *The paideia proposal, an educational manifesto.* New York: Macmillan Publishing Co.

Ahern, Elizabeth Lowe. (2006) *The Pilates method and Ballet Technique: Applications in the Dance Studio.* The Journal of Dance Education, vol. 6, no. 3, 2006.

American Psychological Association Code of Ethics. http://www.apa.org/ethics/code.html.

American Society of Exercise Physiologists Code of Ethics. http://faculty.css.edu/tboone2/asep/ethics.htm.

Answers.com. Definition of Periodic Table of Elements. http://www.answers.com/topic/periodic-table.

Aries, Philippe; Duby, Andre and Veyne, Paul. (1987) *A history of private life, volume i, from pagan rome to byzantium (history of private life. Cambridge, Massachusetts:* Harvard University Press.

Asthma Care Ireland. (2008) *Breath hold as a determinant of performance in sports.* http://www.asthmacare.ie.

Chang, Aileen. (2008) Consultant.
Arlington, Virginia.
achang429@yahoo.com.

Crittenden, Jack. (2008) *Civic education.* Stanford Encyclopedia of Philosophy online. http://plato.stanford.edu/entries/civic-education/.

Fiasca, Peter. (1992) "A Research Study on Anxiety & Movement." Doctoral dissertation.

Franklin, Eric. (1996) *Inner focus, outer strength.* Hightstown, NJ: Princeton Book Company.

Friedman, P., and Eisen, G. (2005) *The Pilates method of physical and mental conditioning.* New York: Viking Penguin Publishers.

Franks, Julie. (2008) Editorial Consultant. jf642@columbia.edu.

Galliano, Siri. (2008) Consultant. Live Art Pilates. 10524 W. Pico Boulevard, Suite 218, Los Angeles, California, 90064. 1.310.963.3683. www.liveartpilates.com • liveartpilates@earthlink.net.

Holy Bible, The: King James Version. (2007) Hendrickson Publishers.

Horney, Karen. (1950) *Neurosis and human growth.* New York: W.W. Norton Company.

Horney, Karen. (1945) *Our inner conflicts.* New York: W.W. Norton Company.

I ching, or the book of changes. (1979) Princeton, NJ: Princeton University Press.

IDEA Health and Fitness Association Code of Ethics. http://www.ideafit.com/code_ethics.asp.

References

Jaeger, Werner. (1979) *Paideia, the ideals of Greek culture.*
New York: Oxford University Press.

Mayers, Lester B., and Rundell, Kenneth W. (2008)
"Exercise-Induced Asthma," *American College of Sports Medicine.*
www.acsm.org.

MedLine. (2008) Definition of rapid shallow breathing.
U.S. National Institutes of Health Medical Dictionary.
www.nlm.nih.gov/medlineplus/ency/article/007198.htm.

Nagel, R., Frey, R., and Betz, D.C. (2007) *Digestive system to the skeleton.* Farmington Hills, MI.

Pilates, J.H., and Miller, J.M. (2000) *Return to life through contrology.* In *The complete writings of Joseph H. Pilates.*
Editors: Gallagher, Sean P., Kryzanowska, Romana.
Philadelphia: BainBridge Books.

Pilates, J.H., and Miller, J.M. (2000) *Your health: A Corrective System of Exercising that Revolutionizes the Entire Field of Physical Education.* In *The complete writings of Joseph H. Pilates.*
Editors: Gallagher, Sean P., Kryzanowska,
Romana. Philadelphia: BainBridge Books.

Siegle, L. (2005) *The encyclopedia of muscle and skeletal systems and disorders.* Chicago: Facts On File Publishers.

Sivananda, Sri Swami. (Buddhist date 5,000.11.71.)
Science of yoga, Vol. I Durban, South Africa: Sivananda Press.

Suzuki, D. T., Fromm, E., and De Martino, R. (1970) *Zen Buddhism and psychoanalysis.* New York: Grove Press.

Tzu, Lao. (1997) *Tao te ching.* London: Vintage Publishers.

Ungaro, Alycea. (2008) Consultant. Real Pilates. 177 Duane Street, New York, NY 10013. 212.625.0777. www.realpilatesnyc.com • info@realpilatesnyc.com.

West, John B. (2000) *Respiratory physiology: the essentials,* sixth edition. Baltimore: Lippincott Williams & Wilkins Publishers.

Weinberg, George. (1985) *The heart of psychotherapy.* New York: St. Martin's Press.

Whipp, B.J. (2008) "Breathing During Exercise." www.answers.com.

Whitacre, Paula Tarnapol. (2008) Editorial Consultant. www.fullcircle.org • ptw@fullcircle.org.

Appendix

The Academy Directory
www.ClassicalPilates.net

The worldwide Academy Directory lists over 1,000 professionals who completed comprehensive training with the most distinguished, traditional 1st & 2nd generation instructors whose training lineage comes directly from Joseph & Clara Pilates. These instructors can be found at *www.classicalpilates.net* on the "Academy Directory" webpage. You can also find the best teacher-training programs on the "Training" webpage.

> What is unique about the worldwide Academy Directory of traditionalists on the *Pure Classical Pilates* website?

- It includes the most comprehensively trained, professionally experienced practitioners of Pure Classical Pilates in the world.
- Membership is free. There are no dues or payments that support a hierarchical organization seeking to establish policy or funding. There is no vested interest other than to help preserve and promote Joseph Pilates' traditional method and the instructors who carry on his work.

- Membership is based upon direct traditional training lineage from Joseph & Clara Pilates.
- Membership requires completion of traditional 600–1,000+ apprenticeship hours from an instructor who is currently listed in the Academy Directory.
- There is a wonderful opportunity to network with like-minded colleagues in the traditional method.
- It is a great referral source for students who travel and would like to take lessons while vacationing or working on the road.

A Pure Classical Collection:
The Principles Come to Life on DVD

Caution
- *These DVDs are not intended for treatment of any injuries.*
- *Do not use as a replacement for medical care.*
- *Always obtain a physician's advice before starting any physical fitness program.*

The collection of **Classical Pilates Technique** DVDs is a glossary of historically accurate movement vocabulary, yet these DVDs are far from complete! Pure Classical Pilates has an infinite number of subtleties and variations that traditionalists should continue to document in new DVDs, books, research articles and other media. We will probably need decades of work to record the breadth and depth of Joseph Pilates' traditional method. Even after decades of filming and research, however, it will be impossible to capture every aspect of the traditional method. We can continue to make progress, however, toward a more complete understanding of the work.

The set of six *Classical Pilates Technique* DVDs has limitations, but it is still useful for reference material or instruction. To be sure, DVDs should only be used as a secondary learning source. It is always best to study with a traditional instructor listed in the Academy Directory.

Although Pure Classical Pilates is an intrinsically communicative and cooperative activity requiring hands-on physical contact, there is a relevant place for filming correct articulation and refinement of each exercise, as well as proper dynamics and smooth transitions. It's also inspiring to see the full-range of exercises in the traditional system.

If students or teachers have only been exposed to basic-intermediate exercises (or workouts), how is it possible for them to be inspired to learn and move toward goals beyond their current level? Technique, in this case, is *not* simply performing exercises; instead, it refers to wholeheartedly incorporating aspects of mind, body, spirit and imagination to support one's evolution toward deepening self-knowledge and expanding athletic artistry. The true nature and aim of Joseph Pilates' traditional method is nothing less than becoming a more complete human being.

If an individual does not live near a traditional instructor, or they don't have time or money for lessons, DVD instruction can be better than nothing *if* the viewer works safely, conservatively, and with common sense. My hope is that viewers will be inspired to find a highly qualified instructor in the Academy Directory and study Pure Classical Pilates.

Classical Pilates Technique DVDs demonstrate a progression of safe and effective workouts for the entire mind and body that tone your muscles and uplift the spirit, while remaining true to Joseph Pilates' pure classical form. *Classical Pilates Technique* DVDs serve as the instructional "how-to" companion of this book. By producing and offering these educational tools to the market, I feel deeply thankful to play a role in the preservation of Joseph Pilates' philosophy and technique. The DVD collection includes:

- *Classical Pilates Technique with Consideration of the Neck & Back*

- This DVD contains a full Pre-Pilates section, as well as three complete Classical Pilates modified Mat levels, to help facilitate safety and stability of the neck and back while you enjoy your refreshing workouts. Another goal of this program is to help you safely increase strength, stamina, coordination and flexibility for the entire body.

- *Classical Pilates Technique:*
  Exercises for Kids & Young Adults

- This DVD demonstrates a wonderful curriculum of safe and effective Classical Pilates exercises for children ages 5-12, and workouts for young adults ages 13-17, which helps improve: Personal Body

Image, Mental Concentration, Injury Prevention, Strength & Flexibility, Weight Management, Self-Esteem & Confidence, Coordination & Balance.

- *Classical Pilates Technique:*
  The Complete Mat Workout Series

- This top-selling technique video exhibits the following levels: Modified-Basic, Basic, Intermediate, Advanced, and Super-Advanced workouts. All workouts demonstrate the purely classical forms of Joseph Pilates' method and are performed in real time with flowing movement, technical clarity, and rhythm. As each exercise is presented, the name and number of repetitions are shown on screen.

- *Classical Pilates Technique:*
  The Complete Universal Reformer Series

- This exciting, high-quality 3-hour, 2-DVD technique video demonstrates all new workouts at every level (Introductory-Basic, Basic, Intermediate, Advanced, Super-Advanced, Archival) and includes a wide range of rarely seen or practiced exercises from Joseph Pilates' archives.

- *Classical Pilates Technique:*
  The Complete Magic Circle Mat Series &
  Reformer Mat Workout

- This DVD is a very exciting combination of Joseph Pilates' classical Mat workouts at every level with his Magic Circle apparatus. Joseph Pilates invented the Magic Circle back in the 1920s to help people feel their muscles more deeply and to engage the Powerhouse more completely. On this DVD, too, is the rarely seen Super-Advanced Reformer Mat Workout. This fantastic workout demonstrates the complete Super-Advanced Universal Reformer series of exercises on the Mat.

- *Classical Pilates Technique: Studio Apparatus Series (2-DVD set)*

- This 4-hour, 2-DVD set exhibits the most diverse and extensive single-source compilation of exercises ever filmed on the following studio apparatus designed by Joseph Pilates: Cadillac, High Chair, Wunda Chair, Low Barrel, Spine Corrector Barrel, High Barrel, Pedi-Pole, Magic Circle, Foot Corrector, Sand Bag, The Wall, Toe Corrector, Magic Square, and Push Up Handles. All exercises demonstrate the purely classical forms of Joseph Pilates' method and are performed in real time with flowing movement, technical clarity, and rhythm. As each exercise is presented, the name and number of repetitions are shown on screen.

PETER FIASCA is from Southern California and began the Pilates method during 1988 at Wee-Tai Hom's studio in New York City. In 1997 he began training with master instructor Romana Kryzanowska at Drago's Gym. He was certified by Romana in 1998 and continued weekly lessons with her through 2002. Over the years, Peter has sustained his education and training with master teachers Jay Grimes and Kathy Grant, as well as other traditional instructors.

In addition to producing and directing the award-winning Classical Pilates Technique series of six DVDs, Peter has been a guest instructor at numerous training centers throughout the U.S. as well as Europe and South America. Peter demonstrated Pilates, and was a periodic guest co-host on QVC cable television from 1997-2002.

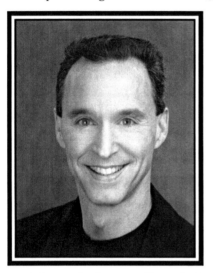

In 2001 Peter demonstrated a Pilates Mat workout taught by Romana Kryzanowska on her first commercial DVD project.

Peter earned a M.A. in developmental psychology and a M.Ed. in psychological counseling at Columbia University then completed his Ph.D. degree in psychology at The Union Institute and was licensed to practice in Pennsylvania. In New York City, Peter worked at The Post Graduate Center for Mental Health, Washington Square Institute and The Karen Horney Clinic. After relocating to Philadelphia in 1993, he worked as a staff psychologist and treatment team coordinator at Girard Medical Center's inpatient and outpatient facilities. From 1997-2001 Peter was a staff psychologist at Abington Memorial Hospital's Creekwood center then opened his own independent psychology practice.

During all this time the Pilates method remained in Peter's body, heart and spirit. In December 2008, he returned to psychology as the associate director of adult outpatient services at CATCH, Inc., in Philadelphia. Yet Peter will continue to teach and study Joseph Pilates' traditional work, devoting himself to the preservation of this extraordinary system of mental and physical conditioning. Consultation services are available upon request: to contact Peter visit the www.ClassicalPilates.net Contact page or call 215.205.8004.

Breinigsville, PA USA
20 October 2009
226172BV00002B/61/P